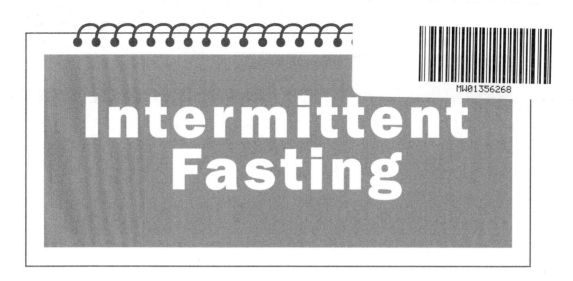

MY DAILY PLANNER

Copyright © 2021 by Blue Book Press
All rights reserved. No part of this publication may be reproduced
or used in any manner whatsoever without the express written permission
of the publisher.

Want a freebie?
Email us at lovelybluebook@gmail.com
Our website:
www.bluebookpress.com

Introduction to the Keto Diet & Intermittent Fasting

Intermittent Fasting and the Keto diet share many of the same health benefits; weight loss, better cognitive function, stabilized blood sugar levels, and lower inflammation. Now then, the question is: should you combine the two for the maximum results?

Let's dive into a few basics concerning the Keto Diet & Intermittent Fasting. Once you know a little more about these two weight loss methods, you'll see why combining the mentioned two is such a powerful weight loss tool.

Ketogenic Diet

The keto diet is a strict low carb diet that requires you to dramatically decrease your carb intake. This could mean consuming anywhere from 20-50 grams of carbs per day depending on your gender, weight, and activity level.

Limiting your diet to low carb foods and healthy fats leads your body into ketosis which is a metabolic state in which your body burns fat stores for energy rather than glucose.

The Ketogenic Diet Keeps You full for a long time. The high level of healthy fat in the keto diet also makes it much easier to stay full –bellied in a fasted state and eliminates those intense feelings of hunger and cravings throughout the day that are usually the greatest obstacles when trying to lose weight.

You avoid all sugary as well as processed foods on a **ketogenic diet**. Some vegetables and fruits also need to be avoided because of the number of carbs they contain.

Vegetables to avoid on keto: Potatoes, carrots, peas, beets, parsnips, sweet potato, butternut squash, most beans, corn, beets, yams.

Fruits to avoid on keto: Bananas, Mangos, Pears, Apples, Pineapples, Plumps, Dates, Grapes, Oranges, Pomegranates, Nectarines, Peaches, Melons, Tangerines, Figs, Kiwi, Prunes.

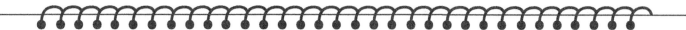

Benefits of Keto Diet:

- Weight Loss
- Appetite Suppressant - You're in more control of your hunger when your body turns to fat stores for energy making Intermittent Fasting easier.
- Type 2 Diabetes Improvements
- Healthy Heart Benefits: Many studies show improved cholesterol figures, lowered blood pressure and, a more balanced heart rate
- Better Focus/Clarity/Understanding

Intermittent Fasting

Intermittent fasting (IF), also known as time-restricted feeding, means eating within a specific daily window of time (feeding period) and fasting outside of that window (fasting period).

Intermittent Fasting is not about starvation. It's not about counting calories, the point is to take control of your hunger, weight loss, activity level, and health. Fasting works for weight loss by allowing your body time to burn off excess fat.

Insulin is the hormone that rules the mentioned process. When we consume, insulin levels rise triggering our body to store sugar and fat. When we fast, insulin levels decrease, which signals our body to burn that stored energy. If you want to lose weight, you have to give your body time to use stored in your organism energy. **That's what Intermittent Fasting does!**

Benefits of Intermittent Fasting

- Weight Loss + Body Fat Loss
- Improved Fat Burning
- Improved Cognitive Function + Mental Clarity
- Improved Lipid Profiles (Better Cholesterol Numbers)
- Lower inflammation
- Better Metabolic Health
- Longevity

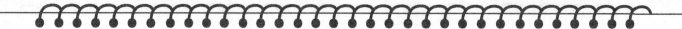

Intermittent Fasting Schedules :

These are popular Intermittent Fasting schedules, but there aren't any rules that say you cannot adapt your own fasting schedule once you learn what works or doesn't work for you! In fact, that's precisely what you ought to do!

16/8 - Doing an 16/8 intermittent fast means that you fast for 16 hours and eat only within an eight-hour window throughout the day, such as from noon to 8 p.m.

18/6 - In this approach you might only eat within a six-hour window (18/6) and a 18 hour fasting time.

23/1 OMAD - Allows a 1-hour eating window and a 23 hour fasting time.

Tips to Get Started:

- Don't start with both methods at once! It takes a few weeks to adjust to a low carb, Ketogenic lifestyle to your organism. Start by getting adapted to the keto diet, then try Intermittent Fasting after you've reached ketosis. If you try both at the same time, you may be setting yourself up for a situation posing a hazard to your health.
- Pick your fasting window: Choose what hours of fasting will be the most appropriate for you. The easiest approach is to have an early dinner and skip your morning breakfast. For example, eating only from 1 p.m. to 9 p.m.
- Have healthy meals during your eating window - the best keto-friendly foods - (max-20 g carbs)
- Eat fatty, satisfying meals. Eating fatty foods will make it a lot easier and sustainable. Keto foods are healthy and make you full, so you won't be hungry during your fasting window.
- Eat Enough: During your eating windows be sure you are eating enough and you feel full. Intermittent Fasting is not aiming at starvation!
- For the first two weeks, you should do light exercise, without overstraining until you know how your body reacts to Intermittent Fasting.
- Stay hydrated make sure you are drinking enough fluids (water) to avoid dehydration!

The Keto diet and Intermittent Fasting is a safe and powerful tool for improving your health as well as increasing your activity levels. If you want to use fasting for ketosis, it's ideal if you do it while following a keto diet.

You will achieve stunning results!

Intermittent Fasting

Fasting Window   **Eating Window**   **Fasting Window**

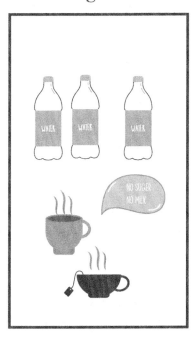
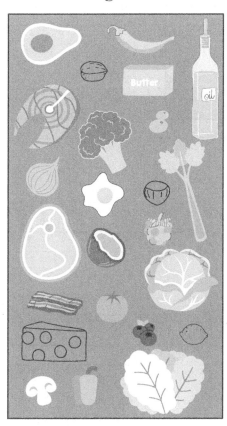
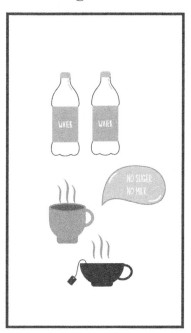

DON'T EAT:

FASTING TIME TRACKER

DATA: _____

MON
Eating Window:

NUMBER OF MEALS:

SUGAR ○ YES ○ NO
COFFEE ○ YES ○ NO
WATER ○ YES ○ NO

FASTING TIME: ○○○○○○○○○○○○○○○○○○○○○○○○ ...... HR

WORKOUT ○ YES ○ NO

TUE
Eating Window:

NUMBER OF MEALS:

SUGAR ○ YES ○ NO
COFFEE ○ YES ○ NO
WATER ○ YES ○ NO

FASTING TIME: ○○○○○○○○○○○○○○○○○○○○○○○○ ...... HR

WORKOUT ○ YES ○ NO

WED
Eating Window:

NUMBER OF MEALS:

SUGAR ○ YES ○ NO
COFFEE ○ YES ○ NO
WATER ○ YES ○ NO

FASTING TIME: ○○○○○○○○○○○○○○○○○○○○○○○○ ...... HR

WORKOUT ○ YES ○ NO

THU
Eating Window:

NUMBER OF MEALS:

SUGAR ○ YES ○ NO
COFFEE ○ YES ○ NO
WATER ○ YES ○ NO

FASTING TIME: ○○○○○○○○○○○○○○○○○○○○○○○○ ...... HR

WORKOUT ○ YES ○ NO

FRI
Eating Window:

NUMBER OF MEALS:

SUGAR ○ YES ○ NO
COFFEE ○ YES ○ NO
WATER ○ YES ○ NO

FASTING TIME: ○○○○○○○○○○○○○○○○○○○○○○○○ ...... HR

WORKOUT ○ YES ○ NO

NOTES & ACCOMPLISHMENT

DATA:		FASTING TIME TRACKER			

SAT
- Eating Window:
- Number of Meals:
- Sugar: ○ YES ○ NO
- Coffee: ○ YES ○ NO
- Water: ○ YES ○ NO
- Fasting Time: ___ HR
- Workout: ○ YES ○ NO

SUN
- Eating Window:
- Number of Meals:
- Sugar: ○ YES ○ NO
- Coffee: ○ YES ○ NO
- Water: ○ YES ○ NO
- Fasting Time: ___ HR
- Workout: ○ YES ○ NO

ENERGY LEVEL

SUN	MON	TUE	WED	THU	FRI	SAT

OBSERVATIONS - HOW I FEEL

MY GOAL THIS WEEK

MEASUREMENT:

CHEST............... WAIST............... HIPS...............

WEIGHT:

FASTING TIME TRACKER

DATA:

MON
- Eating Window:
- NUMBER OF MEALS:
- SUGAR: ○ YES ○ NO
- COFFEE: ○ YES ○ NO
- WATER: ○ YES ○ NO
- FASTING TIME: .... HR
- WORKOUT: ○ YES ○ NO

TUE
- Eating Window:
- NUMBER OF MEALS:
- SUGAR: ○ YES ○ NO
- COFFEE: ○ YES ○ NO
- WATER: ○ YES ○ NO
- FASTING TIME: .... HR
- WORKOUT: ○ YES ○ NO

WED
- Eating Window:
- NUMBER OF MEALS:
- SUGAR: ○ YES ○ NO
- COFFEE: ○ YES ○ NO
- WATER: ○ YES ○ NO
- FASTING TIME: .... HR
- WORKOUT: ○ YES ○ NO

THU
- Eating Window:
- NUMBER OF MEALS:
- SUGAR: ○ YES ○ NO
- COFFEE: ○ YES ○ NO
- WATER: ○ YES ○ NO
- FASTING TIME: .... HR
- WORKOUT: ○ YES ○ NO

FRI
- Eating Window:
- NUMBER OF MEALS:
- SUGAR: ○ YES ○ NO
- COFFEE: ○ YES ○ NO
- WATER: ○ YES ○ NO
- FASTING TIME: .... HR
- WORKOUT: ○ YES ○ NO

NOTES & ACCOMPLISHMENT

DATA:			FASTING TIME TRACKER			

SAT
- Eating Window:
- Number of Meals:
- Fasting Time: ◯◯◯◯◯◯◯◯◯◯◯◯◯◯◯◯◯◯◯◯◯◯◯◯ HR
- SUGAR ◯ YES ◯ NO
- COFFEE ◯ YES ◯ NO
- WATER ◯ YES ◯ NO
- WORKOUT ◯ YES ◯ NO

SUN
- Eating Window:
- Number of Meals:
- Fasting Time: ◯◯◯◯◯◯◯◯◯◯◯◯◯◯◯◯◯◯◯◯◯◯◯◯ HR
- SUGAR ◯ YES ◯ NO
- COFFEE ◯ YES ◯ NO
- WATER ◯ YES ◯ NO
- WORKOUT ◯ YES ◯ NO

ENERGY LEVEL

😄 🙂 😏 😮 😬 😖

SUN	MON	TUE	WED	THU	FRI	SAT

OBSERVATIONS - HOW I FEEL

MY GOAL THIS WEEK

MEASUREMENT:

CHEST.................... WAIST.................... HIPS....................

WEIGHT:

DATA:		FASTING TIME TRACKER			

		Eating Window	NUMBER OF MEALS	SUGAR ○ YES ○ NO
MON				COFFEE ○ YES ○ NO
				WATER ○ YES ○ NO
	FASTING TIME	○○○○○○○○○○○○○○○○○○○○○○○○ ....HR		WORKOUT ○ YES ○ NO
TUE		Eating Window	NUMBER OF MEALS	SUGAR ○ YES ○ NO
				COFFEE ○ YES ○ NO
				WATER ○ YES ○ NO
	FASTING TIME	○○○○○○○○○○○○○○○○○○○○○○○○ ....HR		WORKOUT ○ YES ○ NO
WED		Eating Window	NUMBER OF MEALS	SUGAR ○ YES ○ NO
				COFFEE ○ YES ○ NO
				WATER ○ YES ○ NO
	FASTING TIME	○○○○○○○○○○○○○○○○○○○○○○○○ ....HR		WORKOUT ○ YES ○ NO
THU		Eating Window	NUMBER OF MEALS	SUGAR ○ YES ○ NO
				COFFEE ○ YES ○ NO
				WATER ○ YES ○ NO
	FASTING TIME	○○○○○○○○○○○○○○○○○○○○○○○○ ....HR		WORKOUT ○ YES ○ NO
FRI		Eating Window	NUMBLR OF MEALS	SUGAR ○ YES ○ NO
				COFFEE ○ YES ○ NO
				WATER ○ YES ○ NO
	FASTING TIME	○○○○○○○○○○○○○○○○○○○○○○○○ ....HR		WORKOUT ○ YES ○ NO

NOTES & ACCOMPLISHMENT

DATA:		**FASTING TIME TRACKER**		

SAT
- Eating Window:
- Number of Meals:
- Sugar: ○ YES ○ NO
- Coffee: ○ YES ○ NO
- Water: ○ YES ○ NO
- Fasting Time: _____ HR
- Workout: ○ YES ○ NO

SUN
- Eating Window:
- Number of Meals:
- Sugar: ○ YES ○ NO
- Coffee: ○ YES ○ NO
- Water: ○ YES ○ NO
- Fasting Time: _____ HR
- Workout: ○ YES ○ NO

ENERGY LEVEL

SUN	MON	TUE	WED	THU	FRI	SAT

OBSERVATIONS - HOW I FEEL

MY GOAL THIS WEEK

MEASUREMENT:

CHEST................... WAIST................... HIPS...................

WEIGHT:

DATA:		FASTING TIME TRACKER			
MON	Eating Window		NUMBER OF MEALS	SUGAR	○ YES ○ NO
				COFFEE	○ YES ○ NO
				WATER	○ YES ○ NO
FASTING TIME	○○○○○○○○○○○○○○○○○○○○○○○○ ....H:R			WORKOUT	○ YES ○ NO
TUE	Eating Window		NUMBER OF MEALS	SUGAR	○ YES ○ NO
				COFFEE	○ YES ○ NO
				WATER	○ YES ○ NO
FASTING TIME	○○○○○○○○○○○○○○○○○○○○○○○○ ....H:R			WORKOUT	○ YES ○ NO
WED	Eating Window		NUMBER OF MEALS	SUGAR	○ YES ○ NO
				COFFEE	○ YES ○ NO
				WATER	○ YES ○ NO
FASTING TIME	○○○○○○○○○○○○○○○○○○○○○○○○ ....H:R			WORKOUT	○ YES ○ NO
THU	Eating Window		NUMBER OF MEALS	SUGAR	○ YES ○ NO
				COFFEE	○ YES ○ NO
				WATER	○ YES ○ NO
FASTING TIME	○○○○○○○○○○○○○○○○○○○○○○○○ ....H:R			WORKOUT	○ YES ○ NO
FRI	Eating Window		NUMBER OF MEALS	SUGAR	○ YES ○ NO
				COFFEE	○ YES ○ NO
				WATER	○ YES ○ NO
FASTING TIME	○○○○○○○○○○○○○○○○○○○○○○○○ ....H:R			WORKOUT	○ YES ○ NO

NOTES & ACCOMPLISHMENT

DATA:		FASTING TIME TRACKER			

SAT

Eating Window	NUMBER OF MEALS	SUGAR ◯ YES ◯ NO
		COFFEE ◯ YES ◯ NO
		WATER ◯ YES ◯ NO

FASTING TIME	◯◯◯◯◯◯◯◯◯◯◯◯◯◯◯◯◯◯◯◯◯◯◯◯ ....HR	WORKOUT ◯ YES ◯ NO

SUN

Eating Window	NUMBER OF MEALS	SUGAR ◯ YES ◯ NO
		COFFEE ◯ YES ◯ NO
		WATER ◯ YES ◯ NO

FASTING TIME	◯◯◯◯◯◯◯◯◯◯◯◯◯◯◯◯◯◯◯◯◯◯◯◯ ....HR	WORKOUT ◯ YES ◯ NO

ENERGY LEVEL

😁 🙂 😏 😮 😁 😖

SUN	MON	TUE	WED	THU	FRI	SAT

OBSERVATIONS - HOW I FEEL

MY GOAL THIS WEEK

MEASUREMENT:	WEIGHT:
CHEST.............WAIST.............HIPS.............	

FASTING TIME TRACKER

DATA:

MON
Eating Window:

NUMBER OF MEALS:

- SUGAR ⚪ YES ⚪ NO
- COFFEE ⚪ YES ⚪ NO
- WATER ⚪ YES ⚪ NO

FASTING TIME: _____ H:R

WORKOUT ⚪ YES ⚪ NO

TUE
Eating Window:

NUMBER OF MEALS:

- SUGAR ⚪ YES ⚪ NO
- COFFEE ⚪ YES ⚪ NO
- WATER ⚪ YES ⚪ NO

FASTING TIME: _____ H:R

WORKOUT ⚪ YES ⚪ NO

WED
Eating Window:

NUMBER OF MEALS:

- SUGAR ⚪ YES ⚪ NO
- COFFEE ⚪ YES ⚪ NO
- WATER ⚪ YES ⚪ NO

FASTING TIME: _____ H:R

WORKOUT ⚪ YES ⚪ NO

THU
Eating Window:

NUMBER OF MEALS:

- SUGAR ⚪ YES ⚪ NO
- COFFEE ⚪ YES ⚪ NO
- WATER ⚪ YES ⚪ NO

FASTING TIME: _____ H:R

WORKOUT ⚪ YES ⚪ NO

FRI
Eating Window:

NUMBER OF MEALS:

- SUGAR ⚪ YES ⚪ NO
- COFFEE ⚪ YES ⚪ NO
- WATER ⚪ YES ⚪ NO

FASTING TIME: _____ H:R

WORKOUT ⚪ YES ⚪ NO

NOTES & ACCOMPLISHMENT

DATA:		FASTING TIME TRACKER			

SAT
- Eating Window
- NUMBER OF MEALS
- SUGAR ○ YES ○ NO
- COFFEE ○ YES ○ NO
- WATER ○ YES ○ NO

FASTING TIME: ○○○○○○○○○○○○○○○○○○○○○○○○ ...HR
WORKOUT ○ YES ○ NO

SUN
- Eating Window
- NUMBER OF MEALS
- SUGAR ○ YES ○ NO
- COFFEE ○ YES ○ NO
- WATER ○ YES ○ NO

FASTING TIME: ○○○○○○○○○○○○○○○○○○○○○○○○ ...HR
WORKOUT ○ YES ○ NO

ENERGY LEVEL

SUN	MON	TUE	WED	THU	FRI	SAT

OBSERVATIONS - HOW I FEEL

MY GOAL THIS WEEK

MEASUREMENT:

CHEST................ WAIST................ HIPS................

WEIGHT:

DATA:	FASTING TIME TRACKER		

MON
Eating Window — NUMBER OF MEALS

SUGAR ○ YES ○ NO
COFFEE ○ YES ○ NO
WATER ○ YES ○ NO

FASTING TIME ○○○○○○○○○○○○○○○○○○○○○○○○ ....HR
WORKOUT ○ YES ○ NO

TUE
Eating Window — NUMBER OF MEALS

SUGAR ○ YES ○ NO
COFFEE ○ YES ○ NO
WATER ○ YES ○ NO

FASTING TIME ○○○○○○○○○○○○○○○○○○○○○○○○ ....HR
WORKOUT ○ YES ○ NO

WED
Eating Window — NUMBER OF MEALS

SUGAR ○ YES ○ NO
COFFEE ○ YES ○ NO
WATER ○ YES ○ NO

FASTING TIME ○○○○○○○○○○○○○○○○○○○○○○○○ ....HR
WORKOUT ○ YES ○ NO

THU
Eating Window — NUMBER OF MEALS

SUGAR ○ YES ○ NO
COFFEE ○ YES ○ NO
WATER ○ YES ○ NO

FASTING TIME ○○○○○○○○○○○○○○○○○○○○○○○○ ....HR
WORKOUT ○ YES ○ NO

FRI
Eating Window — NUMBER OF MEALS

SUGAR ○ YES ○ NO
COFFEE ○ YES ○ NO
WATER ○ YES ○ NO

FASTING TIME ○○○○○○○○○○○○○○○○○○○○○○○○ ....HR
WORKOUT ○ YES ○ NO

NOTES & ACCOMPLISHMENT

DATA:		FASTING TIME TRACKER			

SAT
Eating Window

NUMBER OF MEALS

SUGAR ○ YES ○ NO
COFFEE ○ YES ○ NO
WATER ○ YES ○ NO

FASTING TIME ○○○○○○○○○○○○○○○○○○○○○○○○ H

WORKOUT ○ YES ○ NO

SUN
Eating Window

NUMBER OF MEALS

SUGAR ○ YES ○ NO
COFFEE ○ YES ○ NO
WATER ○ YES ○ NO

FASTING TIME ○○○○○○○○○○○○○○○○○○○○○○○○ H

WORKOUT ○ YES ○ NO

ENERGY LEVEL

SUN	MON	TUE	WED	THU	FRI	SAT

OBSERVATIONS - HOW I FEEL

MY GOAL THIS WEEK

MEASUREMENT:

WEIGHT:

CHEST................ WAIST................ HIPS................

DATA:		FASTING TIME TRACKER			
MON	Eating Window		NUMBER OF MEALS	SUGAR	○ YES ○ NO
				COFFEE	○ YES ○ NO
				WATER	○ YES ○ NO
FASTING TIME	○○○○○○○○○○○○○○○○○○○○○○○○ ....HR			WORKOUT	○ YES ○ NO
TUE	Eating Window		NUMBER OF MEALS	SUGAR	○ YES ○ NO
				COFFEE	○ YES ○ NO
				WATER	○ YES ○ NO
FASTING TIME	○○○○○○○○○○○○○○○○○○○○○○○○ ....HR			WORKOUT	○ YES ○ NO
WED	Eating Window		NUMBER OF MEALS	SUGAR	○ YES ○ NO
				COFFEE	○ YES ○ NO
				WATER	○ YES ○ NO
FASTING TIME	○○○○○○○○○○○○○○○○○○○○○○○○ ....HR			WORKOUT	○ YES ○ NO
THU	Eating Window		NUMBER OF MEALS	SUGAR	○ YES ○ NO
				COFFEE	○ YES ○ NO
				WATER	○ YES ○ NO
FASTING TIME	○○○○○○○○○○○○○○○○○○○○○○○○ ....HR			WORKOUT	○ YES ○ NO
FRI	Eating Window		NUMBER OF MEALS	SUGAR	○ YES ○ NO
				COFFEE	○ YES ○ NO
				WATER	○ YES ○ NO
FASTING TIME	○○○○○○○○○○○○○○○○○○○○○○○○ ....HR			WORKOUT	○ YES ○ NO

NOTES & ACCOMPLISHMENT

DATA:		FASTING TIME TRACKER				

SAT
Eating Window		NUMBER OF MEALS	SUGAR ⊙YES ⊙NO
			COFFEE ⊙YES ⊙NO
			WATER ⊙YES ⊙NO
FASTING TIME	○○○○○○○○○○○○☀○○○○○○○○○○○○○ ...HR		WORKOUT ⊙YES ⊙NO

SUN
Eating Window		NUMBER OF MEALS	SUGAR ⊙YES ⊙NO
			COFFEE ⊙YES ⊙NO
			WATER ⊙YES ⊙NO
FASTING TIME	○○○○○○○○○○○○☀○○○○○○○○○○○○○ ...HR		WORKOUT ⊙YES ⊙NO

ENERGY LEVEL
😄 🙂 😏 😮 😬 😵

SUN	MON	TUE	WED	THU	FRI	SAT

OBSERVATIONS - HOW I FEEL

MY GOAL THIS WEEK

MEASUREMENT:
CHEST.......... WAIST.......... HIPS..........

WEIGHT:

DATA:		FASTING TIME TRACKER				
MON	Eating Window		NUMBER OF MEALS	SUGAR	○ YES ○ NO	
				COFFEE	○ YES ○ NO	
				WATER	○ YES ○ NO	
FASTING TIME	○○○○○○○○○○○○○○○○○○○○○○○○		....HR	WORKOUT	○ YES ○ NO	
TUE	Eating Window		NUMBER OF MEALS	SUGAR	○ YES ○ NO	
				COFFEE	○ YES ○ NO	
				WATER	○ YES ○ NO	
FASTING TIME	○○○○○○○○○○○○○○○○○○○○○○○○		....HR	WORKOUT	○ YES ○ NO	
WED	Eating Window		NUMBER OF MEALS	SUGAR	○ YES ○ NO	
				COFFEE	○ YES ○ NO	
				WATER	○ YES ○ NO	
FASTING TIME	○○○○○○○○○○○○○○○○○○○○○○○○		....HR	WORKOUT	○ YES ○ NO	
THU	Eating Window		NUMBER OF MEALS	SUGAR	○ YES ○ NO	
				COFFEE	○ YES ○ NO	
				WATER	○ YES ○ NO	
FASTING TIME	○○○○○○○○○○○○○○○○○○○○○○○○		....HR	WORKOUT	○ YES ○ NO	
FRI	Eating Window		NUMBER OF MEALS	SUGAR	○ YES ○ NO	
				COFFEE	○ YES ○ NO	
				WATER	○ YES ○ NO	
FASTING TIME	○○○○○○○○○○○○○○○○○○○○○○○○		....HR	WORKOUT	○ YES ○ NO	

NOTES & ACCOMPLISHMENT

DATA:		**FASTING TIME TRACKER**			

SAT
- Eating Window:
- Number of Meals:
- Sugar: ○ YES ○ NO
- Coffee: ○ YES ○ NO
- Water: ○ YES ○ NO
- Fasting Time: .... HR
- Workout: ○ YES ○ NO

SUN
- Eating Window:
- Number of Meals:
- Sugar: ○ YES ○ NO
- Coffee: ○ YES ○ NO
- Water: ○ YES ○ NO
- Fasting Time: .... HR
- Workout: ○ YES ○ NO

ENERGY LEVEL

	SUN	MON	TUE	WED	THU	FRI	SAT

OBSERVATIONS - HOW I FEEL

MY GOAL THIS WEEK

MEASUREMENT:

WEIGHT:

CHEST.................... WAIST.................... HIPS....................

DATA:		FASTING TIME TRACKER			
MON	Eating Window		NUMBER OF MEALS	SUGAR	○ YES ○ NO
				COFFEE	○ YES ○ NO
				WATER	○ YES ○ NO
FASTING TIME	○○○○○○○○○○○○☀○○○○○○○○○○○○ ....HR			WORKOUT	○ YES ○ NO
TUE	Eating Window		NUMBER OF MEALS	SUGAR	○ YES ○ NO
				COFFEE	○ YES ○ NO
				WATER	○ YES ○ NO
FASTING TIME	○○○○○○○○○○○○☀○○○○○○○○○○○○ ....HR			WORKOUT	○ YES ○ NO
WED	Eating Window		NUMBER OF MEALS	SUGAR	○ YES ○ NO
				COFFEE	○ YES ○ NO
				WATER	○ YES ○ NO
FASTING TIME	○○○○○○○○○○○○☀○○○○○○○○○○○○ ....HR			WORKOUT	○ YES ○ NO
THU	Eating Window		NUMBER OF MEALS	SUGAR	○ YES ○ NO
				COFFEE	○ YES ○ NO
				WATER	○ YES ○ NO
FASTING TIME	○○○○○○○○○○○○☀○○○○○○○○○○○○ ....HR			WORKOUT	○ YES ○ NO
FRI	Eating Window		NUMBER OF MEALS	SUGAR	○ YES ○ NO
				COFFEE	○ YES ○ NO
				WATER	○ YES ○ NO
FASTING TIME	○○○○○○○○○○○○☀○○○○○○○○○○○○ ....HR			WORKOUT	○ YES ○ NO

NOTES & ACCOMPLISHMENT

DATA:		**FASTING TIME TRACKER**		

SAT	Eating Window	NUMBER OF MEALS	SUGAR ⚪YES ⚪NO
			COFFEE ⚪YES ⚪NO
			WATER ⚪YES ⚪NO
FASTING TIME	⚪⚪⚪⚪⚪⚪⚪⚪⚪⚪⚪⚪⚪⚪⚪⚪⚪⚪⚪⚪⚪⚪⚪⚪ ....HR		WORKOUT ⚪YES ⚪NO

SUN	Eating Window	NUMBER OF MEALS	SUGAR ⚪YES ⚪NO
			COFFEE ⚪YES ⚪NO
			WATER ⚪YES ⚪NO
FASTING TIME	⚪⚪⚪⚪⚪⚪⚪⚪⚪⚪⚪⚪⚪⚪⚪⚪⚪⚪⚪⚪⚪⚪⚪⚪ ....HR		WORKOUT ⚪YES ⚪NO

ENERGY LEVEL

😊 🙂 😒 😮 😁 😟

	SUN	MON	TUE	WED	THU	FRI	SAT

OBSERVATIONS - HOW I FEEL

MY GOAL THIS WEEK

MEASUREMENT: | WEIGHT:

CHEST.............. WAIST.............. HIPS..............

DATA:		FASTING TIME TRACKER			
MON	Eating Window		NUMBER OF MEALS	SUGAR	○ YES ○ NO
				COFFEE	○ YES ○ NO
				WATER	○ YES ○ NO
FASTING TIME	○○○○○○○○○○○○○○○○○○○○○○○○ ...HR			WORKOUT	○ YES ○ NO
TUE	Eating Window		NUMBER OF MEALS	SUGAR	○ YES ○ NO
				COFFEE	○ YES ○ NO
				WATER	○ YES ○ NO
FASTING TIME	○○○○○○○○○○○○○○○○○○○○○○○○ ...HR			WORKOUT	○ YES ○ NO
WED	Eating Window		NUMBER OF MEALS	SUGAR	○ YES ○ NO
				COFFEE	○ YES ○ NO
				WATER	○ YES ○ NO
FASTING TIME	○○○○○○○○○○○○○○○○○○○○○○○○ ...HR			WORKOUT	○ YES ○ NO
THU	Eating Window		NUMBER OF MEALS	SUGAR	○ YES ○ NO
				COFFEE	○ YES ○ NO
				WATER	○ YES ○ NO
FASTING TIME	○○○○○○○○○○○○○○○○○○○○○○○○ ...HR			WORKOUT	○ YES ○ NO
FRI	Eating Window		NUMBER OF MEALS	SUGAR	○ YES ○ NO
				COFFEE	○ YES ○ NO
				WATER	○ YES ○ NO
FASTING TIME	○○○○○○○○○○○○○○○○○○○○○○○○ ...HR			WORKOUT	○ YES ○ NO

NOTES & ACCOMPLISHMENT

DATA:		FASTING TIME TRACKER			

SAT
- Eating Window:
- NUMBER OF MEALS:
- SUGAR ○ YES ○ NO
- COFFEE ○ YES ○ NO
- WATER ○ YES ○ NO
- FASTING TIME: ○○○○○○○○○○○○○○○○○○○○○○○ HR
- WORKOUT ○ YES ○ NO

SUN
- Eating Window:
- NUMBER OF MEALS:
- SUGAR ○ YES ○ NO
- COFFEE ○ YES ○ NO
- WATER ○ YES ○ NO
- FASTING TIME: ○○○○○○○○○○○○○○○○○○○○○○○ HR
- WORKOUT ○ YES ○ NO

ENERGY LEVEL

SUN	MON	TUE	WED	THU	FRI	SAT

OBSERVATIONS - HOW I FEEL

MY GOAL THIS WEEK

MEASUREMENT:

WEIGHT:

CHEST.................. WAIST.................. HIPS..................

| DATA: | | FASTING TIME TRACKER | | | | |

MON	Eating Window		NUMBER OF MEALS	SUGAR ⭘YES ⭘NO
				COFFEE ⭘YES ⭘NO
				WATER ⭘YES ⭘NO
FASTING TIME	⭕⭕⭕⭕⭕⭕⭕⭕⭕⭕⭕⭕⭕☀⭕⭕⭕⭕⭕⭕⭕⭕⭕⭕	......HR	WORKOUT ⭘YES ⭘NO

TUE	Eating Window		NUMBER OF MEALS	SUGAR ⭘YES ⭘NO
				COFFEE ⭘YES ⭘NO
				WATER ⭘YES ⭘NO
FASTING TIME	⭕⭕⭕⭕⭕⭕⭕⭕⭕⭕⭕⭕☀⭕⭕⭕⭕⭕⭕⭕⭕⭕⭕⭕	......HR	WORKOUT ⭘YES ⭘NO

WED	Eating Window		NUMBER OF MEALS	SUGAR ⭘YES ⭘NO
				COFFEE ⭘YES ⭘NO
				WATER ⭘YES ⭘NO
FASTING TIME	⭕⭕⭕⭕⭕⭕⭕⭕⭕⭕⭕⭕☀⭕⭕⭕⭕⭕⭕⭕⭕⭕⭕⭕	......HR	WORKOUT ⭘YES ⭘NO

THU	Eating Window		NUMBER OF MEALS	SUGAR ⭘YES ⭘NO
				COFFEE ⭘YES ⭘NO
				WATER ⭘YES ⭘NO
FASTING TIME	⭕⭕⭕⭕⭕⭕⭕⭕⭕⭕⭕⭕☀⭕⭕⭕⭕⭕⭕⭕⭕⭕⭕⭕	......HR	WORKOUT ⭘YES ⭘NO

FRI	Eating Window		NUMBER OF MEALS	SUGAR ⭘YES ⭘NO
				COFFEE ⭘YES ⭘NO
				WATER ⭘YES ⭘NO
FASTING TIME	⭕⭕⭕⭕⭕⭕⭕⭕⭕⭕⭕⭕☀⭕⭕⭕⭕⭕⭕⭕⭕⭕⭕⭕	......HR	WORKOUT ⭘YES ⭘NO

NOTES & ACCOMPLISHMENT

DATA:	FASTING TIME TRACKER		

SAT
- Eating Window:
- Number of Meals:
- Sugar: ○ YES ○ NO
- Coffee: ○ YES ○ NO
- Water: ○ YES ○ NO
- Fasting Time: ○○○○○○○○○○○○○○○○○○○○○○○○ ____ HR
- Workout: ○ YES ○ NO

SUN
- Eating Window:
- Number of Meals:
- Sugar: ○ YES ○ NO
- Coffee: ○ YES ○ NO
- Water: ○ YES ○ NO
- Fasting Time: ○○○○○○○○○○○○○○○○○○○○○○○○ ____ HR
- Workout: ○ YES ○ NO

ENERGY LEVEL

	SUN	MON	TUE	WED	THU	FRI	SAT

OBSERVATIONS - HOW I FEEL

MY GOAL THIS WEEK

MEASUREMENT:
CHEST........... WAIST........... HIPS...........

WEIGHT:

DATA:	FASTING TIME TRACKER		

MON	Eating Window	NUMBER OF MEALS	SUGAR ○YES ○NO
			COFFEE ○YES ○NO
			WATER ○YES ○NO
FASTING TIME	○○○○○○○○○○○○○○○○○○○○○○○○ ...HR		WORKOUT ○YES ○NO
TUE	Eating Window	NUMBER OF MEALS	SUGAR ○YES ○NO
			COFFEE ○YES ○NO
			WATER ○YES ○NO
FASTING TIME	○○○○○○○○○○○○○○○○○○○○○○○○ ...HR		WORKOUT ○YES ○NO
WED	Eating Window	NUMBER OF MEALS	SUGAR ○YES ○NO
			COFFEE ○YES ○NO
			WATER ○YES ○NO
FASTING TIME	○○○○○○○○○○○○○○○○○○○○○○○○ ...HR		WORKOUT ○YES ○NO
THU	Eating Window	NUMBER OF MEALS	SUGAR ○YES ○NO
			COFFEE ○YES ○NO
			WATER ○YES ○NO
FASTING TIME	○○○○○○○○○○○○○○○○○○○○○○○○ ...HR		WORKOUT ○YES ○NO
FRI	Eating Window	NUMBER OF MEALS	SUGAR ○YES ○NO
			COFFEE ○YES ○NO
			WATER ○YES ○NO
FASTING TIME	○○○○○○○○○○○○○○○○○○○○○○○○ ...HR		WORKOUT ○YES ○NO

NOTES & ACCOMPLISHMENT

DATA:		FASTING TIME TRACKER			

SAT
- Eating Window:
- NUMBER OF MEALS:
- SUGAR ◯ YES ◯ NO
- COFFEE ◯ YES ◯ NO
- WATER ◯ YES ◯ NO
- FASTING TIME: ___ HR
- WORKOUT ◯ YES ◯ NO

SUN
- Eating Window:
- NUMBER OF MEALS:
- SUGAR ◯ YES ◯ NO
- COFFEE ◯ YES ◯ NO
- WATER ◯ YES ◯ NO
- FASTING TIME: ___ HR
- WORKOUT ◯ YES ◯ NO

ENERGY LEVEL

SUN	MON	TUE	WED	THU	FRI	SAT

OBSERVATIONS - HOW I FEEL

MY GOAL THIS WEEK

MEASUREMENT:

CHEST............ WAIST............ HIPS............

WEIGHT:

FASTING TIME TRACKER

DATA:

MON
Eating Window

NUMBER OF MEALS

- SUGAR ○ YES ○ NO
- COFFEE ○ YES ○ NO
- WATER ○ YES ○ NO

FASTING TIME ....HR — WORKOUT ○ YES ○ NO

TUE
Eating Window

NUMBER OF MEALS

- SUGAR ○ YES ○ NO
- COFFEE ○ YES ○ NO
- WATER ○ YES ○ NO

FASTING TIME ....HR — WORKOUT ○ YES ○ NO

WED
Eating Window

NUMBER OF MEALS

- SUGAR ○ YES ○ NO
- COFFEE ○ YES ○ NO
- WATER ○ YES ○ NO

FASTING TIME ....HR — WORKOUT ○ YES ○ NO

THU
Eating Window

NUMBER OF MEALS

- SUGAR ○ YES ○ NO
- COFFEE ○ YES ○ NO
- WATER ○ YES ○ NO

FASTING TIME ....HR — WORKOUT ○ YES ○ NO

FRI
Eating Window

NUMBER OF MEALS

- SUGAR ○ YES ○ NO
- COFFEE ○ YES ○ NO
- WATER ○ YES ○ NO

FASTING TIME ....HR — WORKOUT ○ YES ○ NO

NOTES & ACCOMPLISHMENT

DATA:		FASTING TIME TRACKER			

SAT
- Eating Window:
- Number of Meals:
- Sugar: ○ YES ○ NO
- Coffee: ○ YES ○ NO
- Water: ○ YES ○ NO
- Fasting Time: ___ HR
- Workout: ○ YES ○ NO

SUN
- Eating Window:
- Number of Meals:
- Sugar: ○ YES ○ NO
- Coffee: ○ YES ○ NO
- Water: ○ YES ○ NO
- Fasting Time: ___ HR
- Workout: ○ YES ○ NO

ENERGY LEVEL

SUN	MON	TUE	WED	THU	FRI	SAT

OBSERVATIONS - HOW I FEEL

MY GOAL THIS WEEK

MEASUREMENT:

WEIGHT:

CHEST............ WAIST............ HIPS............

DATA:		FASTING TIME TRACKER			
MON	Eating Window		NUMBER OF MEALS	SUGAR ○YES ○NO	
				COFFEE ○YES ○NO	
				WATER ○YES ○NO	
FASTING TIME	○○○○○○○○○○○○○○○○○○○○○○○○ ....H.R			WORKOUT ○YES ○NO	
TUE	Eating Window		NUMBER OF MEALS	SUGAR ○YES ○NO	
				COFFEE ○YES ○NO	
				WATER ○YES ○NO	
FASTING TIME	○○○○○○○○○○○○○○○○○○○○○○○○ ....H.R			WORKOUT ○YES ○NO	
WED	Eating Window		NUMBER OF MEALS	SUGAR ○YES ○NO	
				COFFEE ○YES ○NO	
				WATER ○YES ○NO	
FASTING TIME	○○○○○○○○○○○○○○○○○○○○○○○○ ....H.R			WORKOUT ○YES ○NO	
THU	Eating Window		NUMBER OF MEALS	SUGAR ○YES ○NO	
				COFFEE ○YES ○NO	
				WATER ○YES ○NO	
FASTING TIME	○○○○○○○○○○○○○○○○○○○○○○○○ ....H.R			WORKOUT ○YES ○NO	
FRI	Eating Window		NUMBER OF MEALS	SUGAR ○YES ○NO	
				COFFEE ○YES ○NO	
				WATER ○YES ○NO	
FASTING TIME	○○○○○○○○○○○○○○○○○○○○○○○○ ....H.R			WORKOUT ○YES ○NO	

NOTES & ACCOMPLISHMENT

| DATA: | | FASTING TIME TRACKER | | | | |

SAT
- Eating Window
- NUMBER OF MEALS
- SUGAR ◯ YES ◯ NO
- COFFEE ◯ YES ◯ NO
- WATER ◯ YES ◯ NO

FASTING TIME ....HR WORKOUT ◯ YES ◯ NO

SUN
- Eating Window
- NUMBER OF MEALS
- SUGAR ◯ YES ◯ NO
- COFFEE ◯ YES ◯ NO
- WATER ◯ YES ◯ NO

FASTING TIME ....HR WORKOUT ◯ YES ◯ NO

ENERGY LEVEL

SUN	MON	TUE	WED	THU	FRI	SAT

OBSERVATIONS - HOW I FEEL

MY GOAL THIS WEEK

MEASUREMENT:	WEIGHT:
CHEST................WAIST................HIPS................	

FASTING TIME TRACKER

DATA:

MON
- Eating Window:
- NUMBER OF MEALS:
- SUGAR ○ YES ○ NO
- COFFEE ○ YES ○ NO
- WATER ○ YES ○ NO
- FASTING TIME: ____ HR
- WORKOUT ○ YES ○ NO

TUE
- Eating Window:
- NUMBER OF MEALS:
- SUGAR ○ YES ○ NO
- COFFEE ○ YES ○ NO
- WATER ○ YES ○ NO
- FASTING TIME: ____ HR
- WORKOUT ○ YES ○ NO

WED
- Eating Window:
- NUMBER OF MEALS:
- SUGAR ○ YES ○ NO
- COFFEE ○ YES ○ NO
- WATER ○ YES ○ NO
- FASTING TIME: ____ HR
- WORKOUT ○ YES ○ NO

THU
- Eating Window:
- NUMBER OF MEALS:
- SUGAR ○ YES ○ NO
- COFFEE ○ YES ○ NO
- WATER ○ YES ○ NO
- FASTING TIME: ____ HR
- WORKOUT ○ YES ○ NO

FRI
- Eating Window:
- NUMBER OF MEALS:
- SUGAR ○ YES ○ NO
- COFFEE ○ YES ○ NO
- WATER ○ YES ○ NO
- FASTING TIME: ____ HR
- WORKOUT ○ YES ○ NO

NOTES & ACCOMPLISHMENT

DATA:	FASTING TIME TRACKER			

SAT
- Eating Window:
- NUMBER OF MEALS:
- SUGAR: ○ YES ○ NO
- COFFEE: ○ YES ○ NO
- WATER: ○ YES ○ NO
- FASTING TIME: .... HR
- WORKOUT: ○ YES ○ NO

SUN
- Eating Window:
- NUMBER OF MEALS:
- SUGAR: ○ YES ○ NO
- COFFEE: ○ YES ○ NO
- WATER: ○ YES ○ NO
- FASTING TIME: .... HR
- WORKOUT: ○ YES ○ NO

ENERGY LEVEL

SUN	MON	TUE	WED	THU	FRI	SAT

OBSERVATIONS - HOW I FEEL

MY GOAL THIS WEEK

MEASUREMENT:
CHEST................ WAIST................ HIPS................

WEIGHT:

DATA:		FASTING TIME TRACKER				
MON	Eating Window		NUMBER OF MEALS	SUGAR	○ YES	○ NO
				COFFEE	○ YES	○ NO
				WATER	○ YES	○ NO
FASTING TIME	○○○○○○○○○○○○○○○○○○○○○○○○ ....HR			WORKOUT	○ YES	○ NO
TUE	Eating Window		NUMBER OF MEALS	SUGAR	○ YES	○ NO
				COFFEE	○ YES	○ NO
				WATER	○ YES	○ NO
FASTING TIME	○○○○○○○○○○○○○○○○○○○○○○○○ ....HR			WORKOUT	○ YES	○ NO
WED	Eating Window		NUMBER OF MEALS	SUGAR	○ YES	○ NO
				COFFEE	○ YES	○ NO
				WATER	○ YES	○ NO
FASTING TIME	○○○○○○○○○○○○○○○○○○○○○○○○ ....HR			WORKOUT	○ YES	○ NO
THU	Eating Window		NUMBER OF MEALS	SUGAR	○ YES	○ NO
				COFFEE	○ YES	○ NO
				WATER	○ YES	○ NO
FASTING TIME	○○○○○○○○○○○○○○○○○○○○○○○○ ....HR			WORKOUT	○ YES	○ NO
FRI	Eating Window		NUMBER OF MEALS	SUGAR	○ YES	○ NO
				COFFEE	○ YES	○ NO
				WATER	○ YES	○ NO
FASTING TIME	○○○○○○○○○○○○○○○○○○○○○○○○ ....HR			WORKOUT	○ YES	○ NO

NOTES & ACCOMPLISHMENT

DATA:	FASTING TIME TRACKER		

	Eating Window	NUMBER OF MEALS	SUGAR ○ YES ○ NO
SAT			COFFEE ○ YES ○ NO
			WATER ○ YES ○ NO
FASTING TIME	○○○○○○○○○○○○○○○○○○○○○○○○ ....HR		WORKOUT ○ YES ○ NO
	Eating Window	NUMBER OF MEALS	SUGAR ○ YES ○ NO
SUN			COFFEE ○ YES ○ NO
			WATER ○ YES ○ NO
FASTING TIME	○○○○○○○○○○○○○○○○○○○○○○○○ ....HR		WORKOUT ○ YES ○ NO

ENERGY LEVEL

SUN	MON	TUE	WED	THU	FRI	SAT

OBSERVATIONS - HOW I FEEL

MY GOAL THIS WEEK

MEASUREMENT:

WEIGHT:

CHEST............... WAIST............... HIPS...............

DATA:	FASTING TIME TRACKER		

MON
Eating Window — NUMBER OF MEALS
- SUGAR ○ YES ○ NO
- COFFEE ○ YES ○ NO
- WATER ○ YES ○ NO

FASTING TIME ....HR — WORKOUT ○ YES ○ NO

TUE
Eating Window — NUMBER OF MEALS
- SUGAR ○ YES ○ NO
- COFFEE ○ YES ○ NO
- WATER ○ YES ○ NO

FASTING TIME ....HR — WORKOUT ○ YES ○ NO

WED
Eating Window — NUMBER OF MEALS
- SUGAR ○ YES ○ NO
- COFFEE ○ YES ○ NO
- WATER ○ YES ○ NO

FASTING TIME ....HR — WORKOUT ○ YES ○ NO

THU
Eating Window — NUMBER OF MEALS
- SUGAR ○ YES ○ NO
- COFFEE ○ YES ○ NO
- WATER ○ YES ○ NO

FASTING TIME ....HR — WORKOUT ○ YES ○ NO

FRI
Eating Window — NUMBER OF MEALS
- SUGAR ○ YES ○ NO
- COFFEE ○ YES ○ NO
- WATER ○ YES ○ NO

FASTING TIME ....HR — WORKOUT ○ YES ○ NO

NOTES & ACCOMPLISHMENT

DATA:		FASTING TIME TRACKER			

SAT
- Eating Window:
- Number of Meals:
- Sugar: ○ YES ○ NO
- Coffee: ○ YES ○ NO
- Water: ○ YES ○ NO
- Fasting Time: ___ HR
- Workout: ○ YES ○ NO

SUN
- Eating Window:
- Number of Meals:
- Sugar: ○ YES ○ NO
- Coffee: ○ YES ○ NO
- Water: ○ YES ○ NO
- Fasting Time: ___ HR
- Workout: ○ YES ○ NO

ENERGY LEVEL

SUN	MON	TUE	WED	THU	FRI	SAT

OBSERVATIONS - HOW I FEEL

MY GOAL THIS WEEK

MEASUREMENT:
CHEST......... WAIST......... HIPS.........

WEIGHT:

DATA:	FASTING TIME TRACKER		

MON	Eating Window	NUMBER OF MEALS	SUGAR ⚪YES ⚪NO
			COFFEE ⚪YES ⚪NO
			WATER ⚪YES ⚪NO
FASTING TIME	⭕⭕⭕⭕⭕⭕⭕⭕⭕⭕⭕⭕☀️⭕⭕⭕⭕⭕⭕⭕⭕⭕⭕⭕ ....HR		WORKOUT ⚪YES ⚪NO

TUE	Eating Window	NUMBER OF MEALS	SUGAR ⚪YES ⚪NO
			COFFEE ⚪YES ⚪NO
			WATER ⚪YES ⚪NO
FASTING TIME	⭕⭕⭕⭕⭕⭕⭕⭕⭕⭕⭕⭕☀️⭕⭕⭕⭕⭕⭕⭕⭕⭕⭕⭕ ....HR		WORKOUT ⚪YES ⚪NO

WED	Eating Window	NUMBER OF MEALS	SUGAR ⚪YES ⚪NO
			COFFEE ⚪YES ⚪NO
			WATER ⚪YES ⚪NO
FASTING TIME	⭕⭕⭕⭕⭕⭕⭕⭕⭕⭕⭕⭕☀️⭕⭕⭕⭕⭕⭕⭕⭕⭕⭕⭕ ....HR		WORKOUT ⚪YES ⚪NO

THU	Eating Window	NUMBER OF MEALS	SUGAR ⚪YES ⚪NO
			COFFEE ⚪YES ⚪NO
			WATER ⚪YES ⚪NO
FASTING TIME	⭕⭕⭕⭕⭕⭕⭕⭕⭕⭕⭕⭕☀️⭕⭕⭕⭕⭕⭕⭕⭕⭕⭕⭕ ....HR		WORKOUT ⚪YES ⚪NO

FRI	Eating Window	NUMBER OF MEALS	SUGAR ⚪YES ⚪NO
			COFFEE ⚪YES ⚪NO
			WATER ⚪YES ⚪NO
FASTING TIME	⭕⭕⭕⭕⭕⭕⭕⭕⭕⭕⭕⭕☀️⭕⭕⭕⭕⭕⭕⭕⭕⭕⭕⭕ ....HR		WORKOUT ⚪YES ⚪NO

NOTES & ACCOMPLISHMENT

DATA:		**FASTING TIME TRACKER**			

SAT
Eating Window

NUMBER OF MEALS	SUGAR	○ YES ○ NO
	COFFEE	○ YES ○ NO
	WATER	○ YES ○ NO

FASTING TIME: ○○○○○○○○○○○○○○○○○○○○○○○○ ....HR WORKOUT ○ YES ○ NO

SUN
Eating Window

NUMBER OF MEALS	SUGAR	○ YES ○ NO
	COFFEE	○ YES ○ NO
	WATER	○ YES ○ NO

FASTING TIME: ○○○○○○○○○○○○○○○○○○○○○○○○ ....HR WORKOUT ○ YES ○ NO

ENERGY LEVEL

SUN	MON	TUE	WED	THU	FRI	SAT

OBSERVATIONS - HOW I FEEL

MY GOAL THIS WEEK

MEASUREMENT:

CHEST................ WAIST................ HIPS................

WEIGHT:

DATA:		FASTING TIME TRACKER			

	Eating Window	NUMBER OF MEALS	SUGAR ◯ YES ◯ NO
MON			COFFEE ◯ YES ◯ NO
			WATER ◯ YES ◯ NO
FASTING TIME	◯◯◯◯◯◯◯◯◯◯◯◯◯◯◯◯◯◯◯◯◯◯◯◯ ......:HR		WORKOUT ◯ YES ◯ NO
	Eating Window	NUMBER OF MEALS	SUGAR ◯ YES ◯ NO
TUE			COFFEE ◯ YES ◯ NO
			WATER ◯ YES ◯ NO
FASTING TIME	◯◯◯◯◯◯◯◯◯◯◯◯◯◯◯◯◯◯◯◯◯◯◯◯ ......:HR		WORKOUT ◯ YES ◯ NO
	Eating Window	NUMBER OF MEALS	SUGAR ◯ YES ◯ NO
WED			COFFEE ◯ YES ◯ NO
			WATER ◯ YES ◯ NO
FASTING TIME	◯◯◯◯◯◯◯◯◯◯◯◯◯◯◯◯◯◯◯◯◯◯◯◯ ......:HR		WORKOUT ◯ YES ◯ NO
	Eating Window	NUMBER OF MEALS	SUGAR ◯ YES ◯ NO
THU			COFFEE ◯ YES ◯ NO
			WATER ◯ YES ◯ NO
FASTING TIME	◯◯◯◯◯◯◯◯◯◯◯◯◯◯◯◯◯◯◯◯◯◯◯◯ ......:HR		WORKOUT ◯ YES ◯ NO
	Eating Window	NUMBER OF MEALS	SUGAR ◯ YES ◯ NO
FRI			COFFEE ◯ YES ◯ NO
			WATER ◯ YES ◯ NO
FASTING TIME	◯◯◯◯◯◯◯◯◯◯◯◯◯◯◯◯◯◯◯◯◯◯◯◯ ......:HR		WORKOUT ◯ YES ◯ NO

NOTES & ACCOMPLISHMENT

DATA:		**FASTING TIME TRACKER**			

SAT	Eating Window	NUMBER OF MEALS	SUGAR ○ YES ○ NO
			COFFEE ○ YES ○ NO
			WATER ○ YES ○ NO
FASTING TIME	○○○○○○○○○○○○○○○☼○○○○○○○○○○○○○○ ....HR		WORKOUT ○ YES ○ NO

SUN	Eating Window	NUMBER OF MEALS	SUGAR ○ YES ○ NO
			COFFEE ○ YES ○ NO
			WATER ○ YES ○ NO
FASTING TIME	○○○○○○○○○○○○○○○☼○○○○○○○○○○○○○○ ....HR		WORKOUT ○ YES ○ NO

ENERGY LEVEL

	SUN	MON	TUE	WED	THU	FRI	SAT

OBSERVATIONS - HOW I FEEL

MY GOAL THIS WEEK

MEASUREMENT:

CHEST.............................WAIST..........................HIPS...........................

WEIGHT:

DATA:	FASTING TIME TRACKER		

MON
- Eating Window
- NUMBER OF MEALS
- SUGAR ○ YES ○ NO
- COFFEE ○ YES ○ NO
- WATER ○ YES ○ NO
- FASTING TIME: ○○○○○○○○○○○○○○○○○○○○○○○ ....HR
- WORKOUT ○ YES ○ NO

TUE
- Eating Window
- NUMBER OF MEALS
- SUGAR ○ YES ○ NO
- COFFEE ○ YES ○ NO
- WATER ○ YES ○ NO
- FASTING TIME: ○○○○○○○○○○○○○○○○○○○○○○○ ....HR
- WORKOUT ○ YES ○ NO

WED
- Eating Window
- NUMBER OF MEALS
- SUGAR ○ YES ○ NO
- COFFEE ○ YES ○ NO
- WATER ○ YES ○ NO
- FASTING TIME: ○○○○○○○○○○○○○○○○○○○○○○○ ....HR
- WORKOUT ○ YES ○ NO

THU
- Eating Window
- NUMBER OF MEALS
- SUGAR ○ YES ○ NO
- COFFEE ○ YES ○ NO
- WATER ○ YES ○ NO
- FASTING TIME: ○○○○○○○○○○○○○○○○○○○○○○○ ....HR
- WORKOUT ○ YES ○ NO

FRI
- Eating Window
- NUMBER OF MEALS
- SUGAR ○ YES ○ NO
- COFFEE ○ YES ○ NO
- WATER ○ YES ○ NO
- FASTING TIME: ○○○○○○○○○○○○○○○○○○○○○○○ ....HR
- WORKOUT ○ YES ○ NO

NOTES & ACCOMPLISHMENT

DATA:		FASTING TIME TRACKER			

SAT
- Eating Window:
- NUMBER OF MEALS:
- SUGAR ○ YES ○ NO
- COFFEE ○ YES ○ NO
- WATER ○ YES ○ NO
- FASTING TIME: ....HR
- WORKOUT ○ YES ○ NO

SUN
- Eating Window:
- NUMBER OF MEALS:
- SUGAR ○ YES ○ NO
- COFFEE ○ YES ○ NO
- WATER ○ YES ○ NO
- FASTING TIME: ....HR
- WORKOUT ○ YES ○ NO

ENERGY LEVEL

SUN	MON	TUE	WED	THU	FRI	SAT

OBSERVATIONS - HOW I FEEL

MY GOAL THIS WEEK

MEASUREMENT:

CHEST.................... WAIST.................... HIPS....................

WEIGHT:

DATA:		FASTING TIME TRACKER			
MON	Eating Window		NUMBER OF MEALS	SUGAR	◯ YES ◯ NO
				COFFEE	◯ YES ◯ NO
				WATER	◯ YES ◯ NO
FASTING TIME	◯◯◯◯◯◯◯◯◯◯◯◯☼◯◯◯◯◯◯◯◯◯◯◯ :HR			WORKOUT	◯ YES ◯ NO
TUE	Eating Window		NUMBER OF MEALS	SUGAR	◯ YES ◯ NO
				COFFEE	◯ YES ◯ NO
				WATER	◯ YES ◯ NO
FASTING TIME	◯◯◯◯◯◯◯◯◯◯◯◯☼◯◯◯◯◯◯◯◯◯◯◯ :HR			WORKOUT	◯ YES ◯ NO
WED	Eating Window		NUMBER OF MEALS	SUGAR	◯ YES ◯ NO
				COFFEE	◯ YES ◯ NO
				WATER	◯ YES ◯ NO
FASTING TIME	◯◯◯◯◯◯◯◯◯◯◯◯☼◯◯◯◯◯◯◯◯◯◯◯ :HR			WORKOUT	◯ YES ◯ NO
THU	Eating Window		NUMBER OF MEALS	SUGAR	◯ YES ◯ NO
				COFFEE	◯ YES ◯ NO
				WATER	◯ YES ◯ NO
FASTING TIME	◯◯◯◯◯◯◯◯◯◯◯◯☼◯◯◯◯◯◯◯◯◯◯◯ :HR			WORKOUT	◯ YES ◯ NO
FRI	Eating Window		NUMBER OF MEALS	SUGAR	◯ YES ◯ NO
				COFFEE	◯ YES ◯ NO
				WATER	◯ YES ◯ NO
FASTING TIME	◯◯◯◯◯◯◯◯◯◯◯◯☼◯◯◯◯◯◯◯◯◯◯◯ :HR			WORKOUT	◯ YES ◯ NO

NOTES & ACCOMPLISHMENT

DATA:		FASTING TIME TRACKER			

SAT
- Eating Window:
- Number of Meals:
- Sugar: ○ YES ○ NO
- Coffee: ○ YES ○ NO
- Water: ○ YES ○ NO
- Fasting Time: ....HR
- Workout: ○ YES ○ NO

SUN
- Eating Window:
- Number of Meals:
- Sugar: ○ YES ○ NO
- Coffee: ○ YES ○ NO
- Water: ○ YES ○ NO
- Fasting Time: ....HR
- Workout: ○ YES ○ NO

ENERGY LEVEL

SUN	MON	TUE	WED	THU	FRI	SAT

OBSERVATIONS - HOW I FEEL

MY GOAL THIS WEEK

MEASUREMENT:

CHEST.................. WAIST.................. HIPS..................

WEIGHT:

DATA:		FASTING TIME TRACKER			
MON	Eating Window		NUMBER OF MEALS	SUGAR ◯ YES ◯ NO	
				COFFEE ◯ YES ◯ NO	
				WATER ◯ YES ◯ NO	
FASTING TIME	◯◯◯◯◯◯◯◯◯◯◯◯◯◯◯◯◯◯◯◯◯◯◯◯		....HR	WORKOUT ◯ YES ◯ NO	
TUE	Eating Window		NUMBER OF MEALS	SUGAR ◯ YES ◯ NO	
				COFFEE ◯ YES ◯ NO	
				WATER ◯ YES ◯ NO	
FASTING TIME	◯◯◯◯◯◯◯◯◯◯◯◯◯◯◯◯◯◯◯◯◯◯◯◯		....HR	WORKOUT ◯ YES ◯ NO	
WED	Eating Window		NUMBER OF MEALS	SUGAR ◯ YES ◯ NO	
				COFFEE ◯ YES ◯ NO	
				WATER ◯ YES ◯ NO	
FASTING TIME	◯◯◯◯◯◯◯◯◯◯◯◯◯◯◯◯◯◯◯◯◯◯◯◯		....HR	WORKOUT ◯ YES ◯ NO	
THU	Eating Window		NUMBER OF MEALS	SUGAR ◯ YES ◯ NO	
				COFFEE ◯ YES ◯ NO	
				WATER ◯ YES ◯ NO	
FASTING TIME	◯◯◯◯◯◯◯◯◯◯◯◯◯◯◯◯◯◯◯◯◯◯◯◯		....HR	WORKOUT ◯ YES ◯ NO	
FRI	Eating Window		NUMBER OF MEALS	SUGAR ◯ YES ◯ NO	
				COFFEE ◯ YES ◯ NO	
				WATER ◯ YES ◯ NO	
FASTING TIME	◯◯◯◯◯◯◯◯◯◯◯◯◯◯◯◯◯◯◯◯◯◯◯◯		....HR	WORKOUT ◯ YES ◯ NO	

NOTES & ACCOMPLISHMENT

DATA:		FASTING TIME TRACKER		

SAT
- Eating Window:
- Number of Meals:
- Sugar: ○ YES ○ NO
- Coffee: ○ YES ○ NO
- Water: ○ YES ○ NO
- Fasting Time: ....HR
- Workout: ○ YES ○ NO

SUN
- Eating Window:
- Number of Meals:
- Sugar: ○ YES ○ NO
- Coffee: ○ YES ○ NO
- Water: ○ YES ○ NO
- Fasting Time: ....HR
- Workout: ○ YES ○ NO

ENERGY LEVEL

SUN	MON	TUE	WED	THU	FRI	SAT

OBSERVATIONS - HOW I FEEL

MY GOAL THIS WEEK

MEASUREMENT:

CHEST............... WAIST............... HIPS...............

WEIGHT:

DATA: _____ **FASTING TIME TRACKER**

	Eating Window	NUMBER OF MEALS	SUGAR ○ YES ○ NO
MON			COFFEE ○ YES ○ NO
			WATER ○ YES ○ NO
FASTING TIME	○○○○○○○○○○○○○○○○○○○○○○○○ ....HR		WORKOUT ○ YES ○ NO
	Eating Window	NUMBER OF MEALS	SUGAR ○ YES ○ NO
TUE			COFFEE ○ YES ○ NO
			WATER ○ YES ○ NO
FASTING TIME	○○○○○○○○○○○○○○○○○○○○○○○○ ....HR		WORKOUT ○ YES ○ NO
	Eating Window	NUMBER OF MEALS	SUGAR ○ YES ○ NO
WED			COFFEE ○ YES ○ NO
			WATER ○ YES ○ NO
FASTING TIME	○○○○○○○○○○○○○○○○○○○○○○○○ ....HR		WORKOUT ○ YES ○ NO
	Eating Window	NUMBER OF MEALS	SUGAR ○ YES ○ NO
THU			COFFEE ○ YES ○ NO
			WATER ○ YES ○ NO
FASTING TIME	○○○○○○○○○○○○○○○○○○○○○○○○ ....HR		WORKOUT ○ YES ○ NO
	Eating Window	NUMBER OF MEALS	SUGAR ○ YES ○ NO
FRI			COFFEE ○ YES ○ NO
			WATER ○ YES ○ NO
FASTING TIME	○○○○○○○○○○○○○○○○○○○○○○○○ ....HR		WORKOUT ○ YES ○ NO

NOTES & ACCOMPLISHMENT

DATA:		FASTING TIME TRACKER				

SAT
- Eating Window
- NUMBER OF MEALS
- SUGAR ○ YES ○ NO
- COFFEE ○ YES ○ NO
- WATER ○ YES ○ NO

FASTING TIME: ○○○○○○○○○○○○○○○○○○○○○○○○ ......HR WORKOUT ○ YES ○ NO

SUN
- Eating Window
- NUMBER OF MEALS
- SUGAR ○ YES ○ NO
- COFFEE ○ YES ○ NO
- WATER ○ YES ○ NO

FASTING TIME: ○○○○○○○○○○○○○○○○○○○○○○○○ ......HR WORKOUT ○ YES ○ NO

ENERGY LEVEL

SUN	MON	TUE	WED	THU	FRI	SAT

OBSERVATIONS - HOW I FEEL

MY GOAL THIS WEEK

MEASUREMENT:

CHEST............ WAIST............ HIPS............

WEIGHT:

DATA:		FASTING TIME TRACKER			
MON	Eating Window		NUMBER OF MEALS	SUGAR	◯ YES ◯ NO
				COFFEE	◯ YES ◯ NO
				WATER	◯ YES ◯ NO
FASTING TIME	○○○○○○○○○○○○○○○○○○○○○○○○ ...HR			WORKOUT	◯ YES ◯ NO
TUE	Eating Window		NUMBER OF MEALS	SUGAR	◯ YES ◯ NO
				COFFEE	◯ YES ◯ NO
				WATER	◯ YES ◯ NO
FASTING TIME	○○○○○○○○○○○○○○○○○○○○○○○○ ...HR			WORKOUT	◯ YES ◯ NO
WED	Eating Window		NUMBER OF MEALS	SUGAR	◯ YES ◯ NO
				COFFEE	◯ YES ◯ NO
				WATER	◯ YES ◯ NO
FASTING TIME	○○○○○○○○○○○○○○○○○○○○○○○○ ...HR			WORKOUT	◯ YES ◯ NO
THU	Eating Window		NUMBER OF MEALS	SUGAR	◯ YES ◯ NO
				COFFEE	◯ YES ◯ NO
				WATER	◯ YES ◯ NO
FASTING TIME	○○○○○○○○○○○○○○○○○○○○○○○○ ...HR			WORKOUT	◯ YES ◯ NO
FRI	Eating Window		NUMBER OF MEALS	SUGAR	◯ YES ◯ NO
				COFFEE	◯ YES ◯ NO
				WATER	◯ YES ◯ NO
FASTING TIME	○○○○○○○○○○○○○○○○○○○○○○○○ ...HR			WORKOUT	◯ YES ◯ NO

NOTES & ACCOMPLISHMENT

DATA:		FASTING TIME TRACKER				

SAT	Eating Window	NUMBER OF MEALS	SUGAR ○ YES ○ NO
			COFFEE ○ YES ○ NO
			WATER ○ YES ○ NO
FASTING TIME	○○○○○○○○○○○○○○○○○○○○○○○○ ....HR		WORKOUT ○ YES ○ NO

SUN	Eating Window	NUMBER OF MEALS	SUGAR ○ YES ○ NO
			COFFEE ○ YES ○ NO
			WATER ○ YES ○ NO
FASTING TIME	○○○○○○○○○○○○○○○○○○○○○○○○ ....HR		WORKOUT ○ YES ○ NO

ENERGY LEVEL

	SUN	MON	TUE	WED	THU	FRI	SAT

OBSERVATIONS - HOW I FEEL

MY GOAL THIS WEEK

MEASUREMENT:	WEIGHT:
CHEST............... WAIST............... HIPS...............	

FASTING TIME TRACKER

DATA:

MON
Eating Window

NUMBER OF MEALS

SUGAR ○ YES ○ NO
COFFEE ○ YES ○ NO
WATER ○ YES ○ NO

FASTING TIME ....HR
WORKOUT ○ YES ○ NO

TUE
Eating Window

NUMBER OF MEALS

SUGAR ○ YES ○ NO
COFFEE ○ YES ○ NO
WATER ○ YES ○ NO

FASTING TIME ....HR
WORKOUT ○ YES ○ NO

WED
Eating Window

NUMBER OF MEALS

SUGAR ○ YES ○ NO
COFFEE ○ YES ○ NO
WATER ○ YES ○ NO

FASTING TIME ....HR
WORKOUT ○ YES ○ NO

THU
Eating Window

NUMBER OF MEALS

SUGAR ○ YES ○ NO
COFFEE ○ YES ○ NO
WATER ○ YES ○ NO

FASTING TIME ....HR
WORKOUT ○ YES ○ NO

FRI
Eating Window

NUMBER OF MEALS

SUGAR ○ YES ○ NO
COFFEE ○ YES ○ NO
WATER ○ YES ○ NO

FASTING TIME ....HR
WORKOUT ○ YES ○ NO

NOTES & ACCOMPLISHMENT

DATA:		**FASTING TIME TRACKER**		

SAT
- Eating Window:
- Number of Meals:
- Sugar: ○ YES ○ NO
- Coffee: ○ YES ○ NO
- Water: ○ YES ○ NO
- Fasting Time: ○○○○○○○○○○○○○○○○○○○○○○○○ ......HR
- Workout: ○ YES ○ NO

SUN
- Eating Window:
- Number of Meals:
- Sugar: ○ YES ○ NO
- Coffee: ○ YES ○ NO
- Water: ○ YES ○ NO
- Fasting Time: ○○○○○○○○○○○○○○○○○○○○○○○○ ......HR
- Workout: ○ YES ○ NO

ENERGY LEVEL

SUN	MON	TUE	WED	THU	FRI	SAT

OBSERVATIONS - HOW I FEEL

MY GOAL THIS WEEK

MEASUREMENT:
CHEST............... WAIST............... HIPS...............

WEIGHT:

DATA:		FASTING TIME TRACKER				
MON	Eating Window			NUMBER OF MEALS	SUGAR	○ YES ○ NO
					COFFEE	○ YES ○ NO
					WATER	○ YES ○ NO
FASTING TIME	○○○○○○○○○○○○○○○○○○○○○○○○ ....HR				WORKOUT	○ YES ○ NO
TUE	Eating Window			NUMBER OF MEALS	SUGAR	○ YES ○ NO
					COFFEE	○ YES ○ NO
					WATER	○ YES ○ NO
FASTING TIME	○○○○○○○○○○○○○○○○○○○○○○○○ ....HR				WORKOUT	○ YES ○ NO
WED	Eating Window			NUMBER OF MEALS	SUGAR	○ YES ○ NO
					COFFEE	○ YES ○ NO
					WATER	○ YES ○ NO
FASTING TIME	○○○○○○○○○○○○○○○○○○○○○○○○ ....HR				WORKOUT	○ YES ○ NO
THU	Eating Window			NUMBER OF MEALS	SUGAR	○ YES ○ NO
					COFFEE	○ YES ○ NO
					WATER	○ YES ○ NO
FASTING TIME	○○○○○○○○○○○○○○○○○○○○○○○○ ....HR				WORKOUT	○ YES ○ NO
FRI	Eating Window			NUMBER OF MEALS	SUGAR	○ YES ○ NO
					COFFEE	○ YES ○ NO
					WATER	○ YES ○ NO
FASTING TIME	○○○○○○○○○○○○○○○○○○○○○○○○ ....HR				WORKOUT	○ YES ○ NO

NOTES & ACCOMPLISHMENT

DATA:	FASTING TIME TRACKER			

SAT
- Eating Window:
- NUMBER OF MEALS:
- SUGAR ○ YES ○ NO
- COFFEE ○ YES ○ NO
- WATER ○ YES ○ NO
- FASTING TIME: .... HR
- WORKOUT ○ YES ○ NO

SUN
- Eating Window:
- NUMBER OF MEALS:
- SUGAR ○ YES ○ NO
- COFFEE ○ YES ○ NO
- WATER ○ YES ○ NO
- FASTING TIME: .... HR
- WORKOUT ○ YES ○ NO

ENERGY LEVEL

SUN	MON	TUE	WED	THU	FRI	SAT

OBSERVATIONS - HOW I FEEL

MY GOAL THIS WEEK

MEASUREMENT:

WEIGHT:

CHEST.................. WAIST.................. HIPS..................

FASTING TIME TRACKER

DATA:

MON
- Eating Window:
- Number of Meals:
- Sugar: ○ YES ○ NO
- Coffee: ○ YES ○ NO
- Water: ○ YES ○ NO
- Fasting Time: _____ HR
- Workout: ○ YES ○ NO

TUE
- Eating Window:
- Number of Meals:
- Sugar: ○ YES ○ NO
- Coffee: ○ YES ○ NO
- Water: ○ YES ○ NO
- Fasting Time: _____ HR
- Workout: ○ YES ○ NO

WED
- Eating Window:
- Number of Meals:
- Sugar: ○ YES ○ NO
- Coffee: ○ YES ○ NO
- Water: ○ YES ○ NO
- Fasting Time: _____ HR
- Workout: ○ YES ○ NO

THU
- Eating Window:
- Number of Meals:
- Sugar: ○ YES ○ NO
- Coffee: ○ YES ○ NO
- Water: ○ YES ○ NO
- Fasting Time: _____ HR
- Workout: ○ YES ○ NO

FRI
- Eating Window:
- Number of Meals:
- Sugar: ○ YES ○ NO
- Coffee: ○ YES ○ NO
- Water: ○ YES ○ NO
- Fasting Time: _____ HR
- Workout: ○ YES ○ NO

NOTES & ACCOMPLISHMENT

DATA:		FASTING TIME TRACKER			

SAT
- Eating Window:
- NUMBER OF MEALS:
- SUGAR ○ YES ○ NO
- COFFEE ○ YES ○ NO
- WATER ○ YES ○ NO
- FASTING TIME: ....HR
- WORKOUT ○ YES ○ NO

SUN
- Eating Window:
- NUMBER OF MEALS:
- SUGAR ○ YES ○ NO
- COFFEE ○ YES ○ NO
- WATER ○ YES ○ NO
- FASTING TIME: ....HR
- WORKOUT ○ YES ○ NO

ENERGY LEVEL

SUN	MON	TUE	WED	THU	FRI	SAT

OBSERVATIONS - HOW I FEEL

MY GOAL THIS WEEK

MEASUREMENT:

CHEST.................... WAIST.................... HIPS....................

WEIGHT:

DATA:		FASTING TIME TRACKER			

MON	Eating Window	NUMBER OF MEALS	SUGAR ○YES ○NO
			COFFEE ○YES ○NO
			WATER ○YES ○NO
FASTING TIME	○○○○○○○○○○○○○○○○○○○○○○○○ ....HR		WORKOUT ○YES ○NO

TUE	Eating Window	NUMBER OF MEALS	SUGAR ○YES ○NO
			COFFEE ○YES ○NO
			WATER ○YES ○NO
FASTING TIME	○○○○○○○○○○○○○○○○○○○○○○○○ ....HR		WORKOUT ○YES ○NO

WED	Eating Window	NUMBER OF MEALS	SUGAR ○YES ○NO
			COFFEE ○YES ○NO
			WATER ○YES ○NO
FASTING TIME	○○○○○○○○○○○○○○○○○○○○○○○○ ....HR		WORKOUT ○YES ○NO

THU	Eating Window	NUMBER OF MEALS	SUGAR ○YES ○NO
			COFFEE ○YES ○NO
			WATER ○YES ○NO
FASTING TIME	○○○○○○○○○○○○○○○○○○○○○○○○ ....HR		WORKOUT ○YES ○NO

FRI	Eating Window	NUMBER OF MEALS	SUGAR ○YES ○NO
			COFFEE ○YES ○NO
			WATER ○YES ○NO
FASTING TIME	○○○○○○○○○○○○○○○○○○○○○○○○ ....HR		WORKOUT ○YES ○NO

NOTES & ACCOMPLISHMENT

DATA:		**FASTING TIME TRACKER**			

	Eating Window	NUMBER OF MEALS	SUGAR ○YES ○NO
SAT			COFFEE ○YES ○NO
			WATER ○YES ○NO
FASTING TIME	○○○○○○○○○○○○○○☀○○○○○○○○○○○○○ ....HR		WORKOUT ○YES ○NO

	Eating Window	NUMBER OF MEALS	SUGAR ○YES ○NO
SUN			COFFEE ○YES ○NO
			WATER ○YES ○NO
FASTING TIME	○○○○○○○○○○○○○○☀○○○○○○○○○○○○○ ....HR		WORKOUT ○YES ○NO

ENERGY LEVEL

SUN	MON	TUE	WED	THU	FRI	SAT

OBSERVATIONS - HOW I FEEL

MY GOAL THIS WEEK

MEASUREMENT:

CHEST............... WAIST............... HIPS...............

WEIGHT:

DATA:	FASTING TIME TRACKER		

MON
- Eating Window
- NUMBER OF MEALS
- SUGAR ○ YES ○ NO
- COFFEE ○ YES ○ NO
- WATER ○ YES ○ NO
- FASTING TIME ....HR
- WORKOUT ○ YES ○ NO

TUE
- Eating Window
- NUMBER OF MEALS
- SUGAR ○ YES ○ NO
- COFFEE ○ YES ○ NO
- WATER ○ YES ○ NO
- FASTING TIME ....HR
- WORKOUT ○ YES ○ NO

WED
- Eating Window
- NUMBER OF MEALS
- SUGAR ○ YES ○ NO
- COFFEE ○ YES ○ NO
- WATER ○ YES ○ NO
- FASTING TIME ....HR
- WORKOUT ○ YES ○ NO

THU
- Eating Window
- NUMBER OF MEALS
- SUGAR ○ YES ○ NO
- COFFEE ○ YES ○ NO
- WATER ○ YES ○ NO
- FASTING TIME ....HR
- WORKOUT ○ YES ○ NO

FRI
- Eating Window
- NUMBER OF MEALS
- SUGAR ○ YES ○ NO
- COFFEE ○ YES ○ NO
- WATER ○ YES ○ NO
- FASTING TIME ....HR
- WORKOUT ○ YES ○ NO

NOTES & ACCOMPLISHMENT

DATA:		FASTING TIME TRACKER				

SAT
- Eating Window:
- NUMBER OF MEALS:
- SUGAR: ○ YES ○ NO
- COFFEE: ○ YES ○ NO
- WATER: ○ YES ○ NO
- FASTING TIME: ○○○○○○○○○○○○○○○○○○○○○○○○ ___ HR
- WORKOUT: ○ YES ○ NO

SUN
- Eating Window:
- NUMBER OF MEALS:
- SUGAR: ○ YES ○ NO
- COFFEE: ○ YES ○ NO
- WATER: ○ YES ○ NO
- FASTING TIME: ○○○○○○○○○○○○○○○○○○○○○○○○ ___ HR
- WORKOUT: ○ YES ○ NO

ENERGY LEVEL
😄 🙂 😒 😐 😬 😰

SUN	MON	TUE	WED	THU	FRI	SAT

OBSERVATIONS - HOW I FEEL

MY GOAL THIS WEEK

MEASUREMENT:

CHEST............ WAIST............ HIPS............

WEIGHT:

DATA:		FASTING TIME TRACKER				
MON	Eating Window			NUMBER OF MEALS	SUGAR	⚪ YES ⚪ NO
					COFFEE	⚪ YES ⚪ NO
					WATER	⚪ YES ⚪ NO
FASTING TIME	⚪⚪⚪⚪⚪⚪⚪⚪⚪⚪⚪⚪⚪⚪⚪⚪⚪⚪⚪⚪⚪⚪⚪⚪			....HR	WORKOUT	⚪ YES ⚪ NO
TUE	Eating Window			NUMBER OF MEALS	SUGAR	⚪ YES ⚪ NO
					COFFEE	⚪ YES ⚪ NO
					WATER	⚪ YES ⚪ NO
FASTING TIME	⚪⚪⚪⚪⚪⚪⚪⚪⚪⚪⚪⚪⚪⚪⚪⚪⚪⚪⚪⚪⚪⚪⚪⚪			....HR	WORKOUT	⚪ YES ⚪ NO
WED	Eating Window			NUMBER OF MEALS	SUGAR	⚪ YES ⚪ NO
					COFFEE	⚪ YES ⚪ NO
					WATER	⚪ YES ⚪ NO
FASTING TIME	⚪⚪⚪⚪⚪⚪⚪⚪⚪⚪⚪⚪⚪⚪⚪⚪⚪⚪⚪⚪⚪⚪⚪⚪			....HR	WORKOUT	⚪ YES ⚪ NO
THU	Eating Window			NUMBER OF MEALS	SUGAR	⚪ YES ⚪ NO
					COFFEE	⚪ YES ⚪ NO
					WATER	⚪ YES ⚪ NO
FASTING TIME	⚪⚪⚪⚪⚪⚪⚪⚪⚪⚪⚪⚪⚪⚪⚪⚪⚪⚪⚪⚪⚪⚪⚪⚪			....HR	WORKOUT	⚪ YES ⚪ NO
FRI	Eating Window			NUMBER OF MEALS	SUGAR	⚪ YES ⚪ NO
					COFFEE	⚪ YES ⚪ NO
					WATER	⚪ YES ⚪ NO
FASTING TIME	⚪⚪⚪⚪⚪⚪⚪⚪⚪⚪⚪⚪⚪⚪⚪⚪⚪⚪⚪⚪⚪⚪⚪⚪			....HR	WORKOUT	⚪ YES ⚪ NO

NOTES & ACCOMPLISHMENT

DATA:		FASTING TIME TRACKER			

SAT
- Eating Window
- NUMBER OF MEALS
- SUGAR ○ YES ○ NO
- COFFEE ○ YES ○ NO
- WATER ○ YES ○ NO

FASTING TIME: ○○○○○○○○○○○○○○○☀○○○○○○○○○○○○○○ ......HR WORKOUT ○ YES ○ NO

SUN
- Eating Window
- NUMBER OF MEALS
- SUGAR ○ YES ○ NO
- COFFEE ○ YES ○ NO
- WATER ○ YES ○ NO

FASTING TIME: ○○○○○○○○○○○○○○○☀○○○○○○○○○○○○○○ ......HR WORKOUT ○ YES ○ NO

ENERGY LEVEL

SUN	MON	TUE	WED	THU	FRI	SAT

OBSERVATIONS - HOW I FEEL

MY GOAL THIS WEEK

MEASUREMENT:

CHEST............ WAIST............ HIPS............

WEIGHT:

DATA:		FASTING TIME TRACKER				
MON	Eating Window			NUMBER OF MEALS	SUGAR ○ YES ○ NO	
					COFFEE ○ YES ○ NO	
					WATER ○ YES ○ NO	
FASTING TIME	○○○○○○○○○○○○☼○○○○○○○○○○○○ ....HR				WORKOUT ○ YES ○ NO	
TUE	Eating Window			NUMBER OF MEALS	SUGAR ○ YES ○ NO	
					COFFEE ○ YES ○ NO	
					WATER ○ YES ○ NO	
FASTING TIME	○○○○○○○○○○○○☼○○○○○○○○○○○○ ....HR				WORKOUT ○ YES ○ NO	
WED	Eating Window			NUMBER OF MEALS	SUGAR ○ YES ○ NO	
					COFFEE ○ YES ○ NO	
					WATER ○ YES ○ NO	
FASTING TIME	○○○○○○○○○○○○☼○○○○○○○○○○○○ ....HR				WORKOUT ○ YES ○ NO	
THU	Eating Window			NUMBER OF MEALS	SUGAR ○ YES ○ NO	
					COFFEE ○ YES ○ NO	
					WATER ○ YES ○ NO	
FASTING TIME	○○○○○○○○○○○○☼○○○○○○○○○○○○ ....HR				WORKOUT ○ YES ○ NO	
FRI	Eating Window			NUMBER OF MEALS	SUGAR ○ YES ○ NO	
					COFFEE ○ YES ○ NO	
					WATER ○ YES ○ NO	
FASTING TIME	○○○○○○○○○○○○☼○○○○○○○○○○○○ ....HR				WORKOUT ○ YES ○ NO	

NOTES & ACCOMPLISHMENT

DATA: **FASTING TIME TRACKER**

SAT
- Eating Window:
- NUMBER OF MEALS:
- SUGAR: ○ YES ○ NO
- COFFEE: ○ YES ○ NO
- WATER: ○ YES ○ NO
- FASTING TIME: .... HR
- WORKOUT: ○ YES ○ NO

SUN
- Eating Window:
- NUMBER OF MEALS:
- SUGAR: ○ YES ○ NO
- COFFEE: ○ YES ○ NO
- WATER: ○ YES ○ NO
- FASTING TIME: .... HR
- WORKOUT: ○ YES ○ NO

ENERGY LEVEL

SUN	MON	TUE	WED	THU	FRI	SAT

OBSERVATIONS - HOW I FEEL

MY GOAL THIS WEEK

MEASUREMENT:
CHEST........... WAIST........... HIPS...........

WEIGHT:

DATA:		FASTING TIME TRACKER			
MON	Eating Window		NUMBER OF MEALS	SUGAR ○YES ○NO
				COFFEE ○YES ○NO
				WATER ○YES ○NO
FASTING TIME	○○○○○○○○○○○○○○○○○○○○○○○○ ....HR			WORKOUT ○YES ○NO
TUE	Eating Window		NUMBER OF MEALS	SUGAR ○YES ○NO
				COFFEE ○YES ○NO
				WATER ○YES ○NO
FASTING TIME	○○○○○○○○○○○○○○○○○○○○○○○○ ....HR			WORKOUT ○YES ○NO
WED	Eating Window		NUMBER OF MEALS	SUGAR ○YES ○NO
				COFFEE ○YES ○NO
				WATER ○YES ○NO
FASTING TIME	○○○○○○○○○○○○○○○○○○○○○○○○ ....HR			WORKOUT ○YES ○NO
THU	Eating Window		NUMBER OF MEALS	SUGAR ○YES ○NO
				COFFEE ○YES ○NO
				WATER ○YES ○NO
FASTING TIME	○○○○○○○○○○○○○○○○○○○○○○○○ ....HR			WORKOUT ○YES ○NO
FRI	Eating Window		NUMBER OF MEALS	SUGAR ○YES ○NO
				COFFEE ○YES ○NO
				WATER ○YES ○NO
FASTING TIME	○○○○○○○○○○○○○○○○○○○○○○○○ ....HR			WORKOUT ○YES ○NO

NOTES & ACCOMPLISHMENT

DATA: | **FASTING TIME TRACKER**

SAT
- Eating Window
- NUMBER OF MEALS:
- SUGAR ◯ YES ◯ NO
- COFFEE ◯ YES ◯ NO
- WATER ◯ YES ◯ NO
- FASTING TIME: .... HR
- WORKOUT ◯ YES ◯ NO

SUN
- Eating Window
- NUMBER OF MEALS:
- SUGAR ◯ YES ◯ NO
- COFFEE ◯ YES ◯ NO
- WATER ◯ YES ◯ NO
- FASTING TIME: .... HR
- WORKOUT ◯ YES ◯ NO

ENERGY LEVEL

SUN	MON	TUE	WED	THU	FRI	SAT

OBSERVATIONS - HOW I FEEL

MY GOAL THIS WEEK

MEASUREMENT:
CHEST................ WAIST................ HIPS................

WEIGHT:

DATA:	FASTING TIME TRACKER		

MON
Eating Window | NUMBER OF MEALS | SUGAR ○ YES ○ NO
COFFEE ○ YES ○ NO
WATER ○ YES ○ NO

FASTING TIME ....HR | WORKOUT ○ YES ○ NO

TUE
Eating Window | NUMBER OF MEALS | SUGAR ○ YES ○ NO
COFFEE ○ YES ○ NO
WATER ○ YES ○ NO

FASTING TIME ....HR | WORKOUT ○ YES ○ NO

WED
Eating Window | NUMBER OF MEALS | SUGAR ○ YES ○ NO
COFFEE ○ YES ○ NO
WATER ○ YES ○ NO

FASTING TIME ....HR | WORKOUT ○ YES ○ NO

THU
Eating Window | NUMBER OF MEALS | SUGAR ○ YES ○ NO
COFFEE ○ YES ○ NO
WATER ○ YES ○ NO

FASTING TIME ....HR | WORKOUT ○ YES ○ NO

FRI
Eating Window | NUMBER OF MEALS | SUGAR ○ YES ○ NO
COFFEE ○ YES ○ NO
WATER ○ YES ○ NO

FASTING TIME ....HR | WORKOUT ○ YES ○ NO

NOTES & ACCOMPLISHMENT

DATA:		FASTING TIME TRACKER			

SAT	Eating Window	NUMBER OF MEALS	SUGAR ○YES ○NO
			COFFEE ○YES ○NO
			WATER ○YES ○NO
FASTING TIME	○○○○○○○○○○○○○○○○○○○○○○○○ ....HR		WORKOUT ○YES ○NO

SUN	Eating Window	NUMBER OF MEALS	SUGAR ○YES ○NO
			COFFEE ○YES ○NO
			WATER ○YES ○NO
FASTING TIME	○○○○○○○○○○○○○○○○○○○○○○○○ ....HR		WORKOUT ○YES ○NO

ENERGY LEVEL

😄 🙂 😒 😐 😬 😖

	SUN	MON	TUE	WED	THU	FRI	SAT

OBSERVATIONS - HOW I FEEL

MY GOAL THIS WEEK

MEASUREMENT:

CHEST............ WAIST............ HIPS............

WEIGHT:

DATA:		FASTING TIME TRACKER			
MON	Eating Window		NUMBER OF MEALS	SUGAR	◯ YES ◯ NO
				COFFEE	◯ YES ◯ NO
				WATER	◯ YES ◯ NO
FASTING TIME	◯◯◯◯◯◯◯◯◯◯◯◯◯◯◯◯◯◯◯◯◯◯◯◯		....HR	WORKOUT	◯ YES ◯ NO
TUE	Eating Window		NUMBER OF MEALS	SUGAR	◯ YES ◯ NO
				COFFEE	◯ YES ◯ NO
				WATER	◯ YES ◯ NO
FASTING TIME	◯◯◯◯◯◯◯◯◯◯◯◯◯◯◯◯◯◯◯◯◯◯◯◯		....HR	WORKOUT	◯ YES ◯ NO
WED	Eating Window		NUMBER OF MEALS	SUGAR	◯ YES ◯ NO
				COFFEE	◯ YES ◯ NO
				WATER	◯ YES ◯ NO
FASTING TIME	◯◯◯◯◯◯◯◯◯◯◯◯◯◯◯◯◯◯◯◯◯◯◯◯		....HR	WORKOUT	◯ YES ◯ NO
THU	Eating Window		NUMBER OF MEALS	SUGAR	◯ YES ◯ NO
				COFFEE	◯ YES ◯ NO
				WATER	◯ YES ◯ NO
FASTING TIME	◯◯◯◯◯◯◯◯◯◯◯◯◯◯◯◯◯◯◯◯◯◯◯◯		....HR	WORKOUT	◯ YES ◯ NO
FRI	Eating Window		NUMBER OF MEALS	SUGAR	◯ YES ◯ NO
				COFFEE	◯ YES ◯ NO
				WATER	◯ YES ◯ NO
FASTING TIME	◯◯◯◯◯◯◯◯◯◯◯◯◯◯◯◯◯◯◯◯◯◯◯◯		....HR	WORKOUT	◯ YES ◯ NO

NOTES & ACCOMPLISHMENT

DATA:		FASTING TIME TRACKER			

SAT
- Eating Window:
- Number of Meals:
- Sugar: ⚪ YES ⚪ NO
- Coffee: ⚪ YES ⚪ NO
- Water: ⚪ YES ⚪ NO
- Fasting Time: ....HR
- Workout: ⚪ YES ⚪ NO

SUN
- Eating Window:
- Number of Meals:
- Sugar: ⚪ YES ⚪ NO
- Coffee: ⚪ YES ⚪ NO
- Water: ⚪ YES ⚪ NO
- Fasting Time: ....HR
- Workout: ⚪ YES ⚪ NO

ENERGY LEVEL

SUN	MON	TUE	WED	THU	FRI	SAT

OBSERVATIONS - HOW I FEEL

MY GOAL THIS WEEK

MEASUREMENT:

CHEST.............. WAIST.............. HIPS..............

WEIGHT:

DATA:	FASTING TIME TRACKER		

MON
- Eating Window
- NUMBER OF MEALS
- SUGAR ○ YES ○ NO
- COFFEE ○ YES ○ NO
- WATER ○ YES ○ NO
- FASTING TIME ....HR
- WORKOUT ○ YES ○ NO

TUE
- Eating Window
- NUMBER OF MEALS
- SUGAR ○ YES ○ NO
- COFFEE ○ YES ○ NO
- WATER ○ YES ○ NO
- FASTING TIME ....HR
- WORKOUT ○ YES ○ NO

WED
- Eating Window
- NUMBER OF MEALS
- SUGAR ○ YES ○ NO
- COFFEE ○ YES ○ NO
- WATER ○ YES ○ NO
- FASTING TIME ....HR
- WORKOUT ○ YES ○ NO

THU
- Eating Window
- NUMBER OF MEALS
- SUGAR ○ YES ○ NO
- COFFEE ○ YES ○ NO
- WATER ○ YES ○ NO
- FASTING TIME ....HR
- WORKOUT ○ YES ○ NO

FRI
- Eating Window
- NUMBER OF MEALS
- SUGAR ○ YES ○ NO
- COFFEE ○ YES ○ NO
- WATER ○ YES ○ NO
- FASTING TIME ....HR
- WORKOUT ○ YES ○ NO

NOTES & ACCOMPLISHMENT

DATA:		FASTING TIME TRACKER			

SAT
- Eating Window:
- NUMBER OF MEALS:
- SUGAR: ○ YES ○ NO
- COFFEE: ○ YES ○ NO
- WATER: ○ YES ○ NO

FASTING TIME: ○○○○○○○○○○○○○○○○○○○○○○○○ ......HR — WORKOUT: ○ YES ○ NO

SUN
- Eating Window:
- NUMBER OF MEALS:
- SUGAR: ○ YES ○ NO
- COFFEE: ○ YES ○ NO
- WATER: ○ YES ○ NO

FASTING TIME: ○○○○○○○○○○○○○○○○○○○○○○○○ ......HR — WORKOUT: ○ YES ○ NO

ENERGY LEVEL

SUN	MON	TUE	WED	THU	FRI	SAT

OBSERVATIONS - HOW I FEEL

MY GOAL THIS WEEK

MEASUREMENT:

CHEST.................. WAIST.................. HIPS..................

WEIGHT:

DATA:		FASTING TIME TRACKER				

	Eating Window	NUMBER OF MEALS	SUGAR	○ YES ○ NO
MON			COFFEE	○ YES ○ NO
			WATER	○ YES ○ NO
FASTING TIME	○○○○○○○○○○○○○○○○○○○○○○○○ ....HR		WORKOUT	○ YES ○ NO
	Eating Window	NUMBER OF MEALS	SUGAR	○ YES ○ NO
TUE			COFFEE	○ YES ○ NO
			WATER	○ YES ○ NO
FASTING TIME	○○○○○○○○○○○○○○○○○○○○○○○○ ....HR		WORKOUT	○ YES ○ NO
	Eating Window	NUMBER OF MEALS	SUGAR	○ YES ○ NO
WED			COFFEE	○ YES ○ NO
			WATER	○ YES ○ NO
FASTING TIME	○○○○○○○○○○○○○○○○○○○○○○○○ ....HR		WORKOUT	○ YES ○ NO
	Eating Window	NUMBER OF MEALS	SUGAR	○ YES ○ NO
THU			COFFEE	○ YES ○ NO
			WATER	○ YES ○ NO
FASTING TIME	○○○○○○○○○○○○○○○○○○○○○○○○ ....HR		WORKOUT	○ YES ○ NO
	Eating Window	NUMBER OF MEALS	SUGAR	○ YES ○ NO
FRI			COFFEE	○ YES ○ NO
			WATER	○ YES ○ NO
FASTING TIME	○○○○○○○○○○○○○○○○○○○○○○○○ ....HR		WORKOUT	○ YES ○ NO

NOTES & ACCOMPLISHMENT

DATA:			FASTING TIME TRACKER			
SAT	Eating Window			NUMBER OF MEALS	SUGAR	⚪ YES ⚪ NO
					COFFEE	⚪ YES ⚪ NO
					WATER	⚪ YES ⚪ NO
FASTING TIME	○○○○○○○○○○○○☼○○○○○○○○○○○○			....H.R	WORKOUT	⚪ YES ⚪ NO
SUN	Eating Window			NUMBER OF MEALS	SUGAR	⚪ YES ⚪ NO
					COFFEE	⚪ YES ⚪ NO
					WATER	⚪ YES ⚪ NO
FASTING TIME	○○○○○○○○○○○○☼○○○○○○○○○○○○			....H.R	WORKOUT	⚪ YES ⚪ NO

ENERGY LEVEL

😊 🙂 😒 😮 😁 😟

SUN	MON	TUE	WED	THU	FRI	SAT

OBSERVATIONS - HOW I FEEL

MY GOAL THIS WEEK

MEASUREMENT:

CHEST............... WAIST............... HIPS...............

WEIGHT:

DATA:		FASTING TIME TRACKER				
MON	Eating Window			NUMBER OF MEALS	SUGAR	◯ YES ◯ NO
					COFFEE	◯ YES ◯ NO
					WATER	◯ YES ◯ NO
FASTING TIME	◯◯◯◯◯◯◯◯◯◯◯◯◯◯◯◯◯◯◯◯◯◯◯◯			......HR	WORKOUT	◯ YES ◯ NO
TUE	Eating Window			NUMBER OF MEALS	SUGAR	◯ YES ◯ NO
					COFFEE	◯ YES ◯ NO
					WATER	◯ YES ◯ NO
FASTING TIME	◯◯◯◯◯◯◯◯◯◯◯◯◯◯◯◯◯◯◯◯◯◯◯◯			......HR	WORKOUT	◯ YES ◯ NO
WED	Eating Window			NUMBER OF MEALS	SUGAR	◯ YES ◯ NO
					COFFEE	◯ YES ◯ NO
					WATER	◯ YES ◯ NO
FASTING TIME	◯◯◯◯◯◯◯◯◯◯◯◯◯◯◯◯◯◯◯◯◯◯◯◯			......HR	WORKOUT	◯ YES ◯ NO
THU	Eating Window			NUMBER OF MEALS	SUGAR	◯ YES ◯ NO
					COFFEE	◯ YES ◯ NO
					WATER	◯ YES ◯ NO
FASTING TIME	◯◯◯◯◯◯◯◯◯◯◯◯◯◯◯◯◯◯◯◯◯◯◯◯			......HR	WORKOUT	◯ YES ◯ NO
FRI	Eating Window			NUMBER OF MEALS	SUGAR	◯ YES ◯ NO
					COFFEE	◯ YES ◯ NO
					WATER	◯ YES ◯ NO
FASTING TIME	◯◯◯◯◯◯◯◯◯◯◯◯◯◯◯◯◯◯◯◯◯◯◯◯			......HR	WORKOUT	◯ YES ◯ NO

NOTES & ACCOMPLISHMENT

DATA:		FASTING TIME TRACKER			

SAT
- Eating Window:
- Number of Meals:
- Sugar: ○ YES ○ NO
- Coffee: ○ YES ○ NO
- Water: ○ YES ○ NO
- Fasting Time: .... HR
- Workout: ○ YES ○ NO

SUN
- Eating Window:
- Number of Meals:
- Sugar: ○ YES ○ NO
- Coffee: ○ YES ○ NO
- Water: ○ YES ○ NO
- Fasting Time: .... HR
- Workout: ○ YES ○ NO

ENERGY LEVEL

SUN	MON	TUE	WED	THU	FRI	SAT

OBSERVATIONS - HOW I FEEL

MY GOAL THIS WEEK

MEASUREMENT:
CHEST............... WAIST............... HIPS...............

WEIGHT:

DATA:	FASTING TIME TRACKER			
MON	Eating Window	NUMBER OF MEALS	SUGAR ○ YES ○ NO
			COFFEE ○ YES ○ NO
			WATER ○ YES ○ NO
FASTING TIME	○○○○○○○○○○○○○○○○○○○○○○○○ ......HR	WORKOUT ○ YES ○ NO
TUE	Eating Window	NUMBER OF MEALS	SUGAR ○ YES ○ NO
			COFFEE ○ YES ○ NO
			WATER ○ YES ○ NO
FASTING TIME	○○○○○○○○○○○○○○○○○○○○○○○○ ......HR	WORKOUT ○ YES ○ NO
WED	Eating Window	NUMBER OF MEALS	SUGAR ○ YES ○ NO
			COFFEE ○ YES ○ NO
			WATER ○ YES ○ NO
FASTING TIME	○○○○○○○○○○○○○○○○○○○○○○○○ ......HR	WORKOUT ○ YES ○ NO
THU	Eating Window	NUMBER OF MEALS	SUGAR ○ YES ○ NO
			COFFEE ○ YES ○ NO
			WATER ○ YES ○ NO
FASTING TIME	○○○○○○○○○○○○○○○○○○○○○○○○ ......HR	WORKOUT ○ YES ○ NO
FRI	Eating Window	NUMBER OF MEALS	SUGAR ○ YES ○ NO
			COFFEE ○ YES ○ NO
			WATER ○ YES ○ NO
FASTING TIME	○○○○○○○○○○○○○○○○○○○○○○○○ ......HR	WORKOUT ○ YES ○ NO

NOTES & ACCOMPLISHMENT

DATA:		FASTING TIME TRACKER			

SAT	Eating Window		NUMBER OF MEALS	SUGAR ○ YES ○ NO
				COFFEE ○ YES ○ NO
				WATER ○ YES ○ NO
FASTING TIME	○○○○○○○○○○○○○○○○○○○○○○○○		H.	WORKOUT ○ YES ○ NO

SUN	Eating Window		NUMBER OF MEALS	SUGAR ○ YES ○ NO
				COFFEE ○ YES ○ NO
				WATER ○ YES ○ NO
FASTING TIME	○○○○○○○○○○○○○○○○○○○○○○○○		H.	WORKOUT ○ YES ○ NO

ENERGY LEVEL

SUN	MON	TUE	WED	THU	FRI	SAT

OBSERVATIONS - HOW I FEEL

MY GOAL THIS WEEK

MEASUREMENT:

CHEST.............. WAIST.............. HIPS..............

WEIGHT:

DATA: _____   **FASTING TIME TRACKER**

MON
- Eating Window: _____
- NUMBER OF MEALS: ____
- SUGAR ○ YES ○ NO
- COFFEE ○ YES ○ NO
- WATER ○ YES ○ NO
- FASTING TIME: ○○○○○○○○○○○○○○○○○○○○○○○○ ____ HR
- WORKOUT ○ YES ○ NO

TUE
- Eating Window: _____
- NUMBER OF MEALS: ____
- SUGAR ○ YES ○ NO
- COFFEE ○ YES ○ NO
- WATER ○ YES ○ NO
- FASTING TIME: ○○○○○○○○○○○○○○○○○○○○○○○○ ____ HR
- WORKOUT ○ YES ○ NO

WED
- Eating Window: _____
- NUMBER OF MEALS: ____
- SUGAR ○ YES ○ NO
- COFFEE ○ YES ○ NO
- WATER ○ YES ○ NO
- FASTING TIME: ○○○○○○○○○○○○○○○○○○○○○○○○ ____ HR
- WORKOUT ○ YES ○ NO

THU
- Eating Window: _____
- NUMBER OF MEALS: ____
- SUGAR ○ YES ○ NO
- COFFEE ○ YES ○ NO
- WATER ○ YES ○ NO
- FASTING TIME: ○○○○○○○○○○○○○○○○○○○○○○○○ ____ HR
- WORKOUT ○ YES ○ NO

FRI
- Eating Window: _____
- NUMBER OF MEALS: ____
- SUGAR ○ YES ○ NO
- COFFEE ○ YES ○ NO
- WATER ○ YES ○ NO
- FASTING TIME: ○○○○○○○○○○○○○○○○○○○○○○○○ ____ HR
- WORKOUT ○ YES ○ NO

NOTES & ACCOMPLISHMENT

DATA:		FASTING TIME TRACKER				

SAT
- Eating Window:
- NUMBER OF MEALS:
- SUGAR ◯ YES ◯ NO
- COFFEE ◯ YES ◯ NO
- WATER ◯ YES ◯ NO
- FASTING TIME: ....HR
- WORKOUT ◯ YES ◯ NO

SUN
- Eating Window:
- NUMBER OF MEALS:
- SUGAR ◯ YES ◯ NO
- COFFEE ◯ YES ◯ NO
- WATER ◯ YES ◯ NO
- FASTING TIME: ....HR
- WORKOUT ◯ YES ◯ NO

ENERGY LEVEL

SUN	MON	TUE	WED	THU	FRI	SAT

OBSERVATIONS - HOW I FEEL

MY GOAL THIS WEEK

MEASUREMENT:

CHEST.......... WAIST.......... HIPS..........

WEIGHT:

DATA:	FASTING TIME TRACKER		

MON
Eating Window | NUMBER OF MEALS
SUGAR ○ YES ○ NO
COFFEE ○ YES ○ NO
WATER ○ YES ○ NO

FASTING TIME ○○○○○○○○○○○○○○○○○○○○○○○○ ....HR WORKOUT ○ YES ○ NO

TUE
Eating Window | NUMBER OF MEALS
SUGAR ○ YES ○ NO
COFFEE ○ YES ○ NO
WATER ○ YES ○ NO

FASTING TIME ○○○○○○○○○○○○○○○○○○○○○○○○ ....HR WORKOUT ○ YES ○ NO

WED
Eating Window | NUMBER OF MEALS
SUGAR ○ YES ○ NO
COFFEE ○ YES ○ NO
WATER ○ YES ○ NO

FASTING TIME ○○○○○○○○○○○○○○○○○○○○○○○○ ....HR WORKOUT ○ YES ○ NO

THU
Eating Window | NUMBER OF MEALS
SUGAR ○ YES ○ NO
COFFEE ○ YES ○ NO
WATER ○ YES ○ NO

FASTING TIME ○○○○○○○○○○○○○○○○○○○○○○○○ ....HR WORKOUT ○ YES ○ NO

FRI
Eating Window | NUMBER OF MEALS
SUGAR ○ YES ○ NO
COFFEE ○ YES ○ NO
WATER ○ YES ○ NO

FASTING TIME ○○○○○○○○○○○○○○○○○○○○○○○○ ....HR WORKOUT ○ YES ○ NO

NOTES & ACCOMPLISHMENT

DATA:		FASTING TIME TRACKER		

SAT
- Eating Window
- NUMBER OF MEALS
- SUGAR ◯ YES ◯ NO
- COFFEE ◯ YES ◯ NO
- WATER ◯ YES ◯ NO

FASTING TIME: ○○○○○○○○○○○○☼○○○○○○○○○○○ ......HR
WORKOUT ◯ YES ◯ NO

SUN
- Eating Window
- NUMBER OF MEALS
- SUGAR ◯ YES ◯ NO
- COFFEE ◯ YES ◯ NO
- WATER ◯ YES ◯ NO

FASTING TIME: ○○○○○○○○○○○○☼○○○○○○○○○○○ ......HR
WORKOUT ◯ YES ◯ NO

ENERGY LEVEL

😄 🙂 😒 😮 😁 😟

SUN	MON	TUE	WED	THU	FRI	SAT

OBSERVATIONS - HOW I FEEL

MY GOAL THIS WEEK

MEASUREMENT:

CHEST............ WAIST............ HIPS............

WEIGHT:

DATA:		FASTING TIME TRACKER				
MON	Eating Window			NUMBER OF MEALS	SUGAR	○ YES ○ NO
					COFFEE	○ YES ○ NO
					WATER	○ YES ○ NO
FASTING TIME	○○○○○○○○○○○○○○○○○○○○○○○○ ....HR				WORKOUT	○ YES ○ NO
TUE	Eating Window			NUMBER OF MEALS	SUGAR	○ YES ○ NO
					COFFEE	○ YES ○ NO
					WATER	○ YES ○ NO
FASTING TIME	○○○○○○○○○○○○○○○○○○○○○○○○ ....HR				WORKOUT	○ YES ○ NO
WED	Eating Window			NUMBER OF MEALS	SUGAR	○ YES ○ NO
					COFFEE	○ YES ○ NO
					WATER	○ YES ○ NO
FASTING TIME	○○○○○○○○○○○○○○○○○○○○○○○○ ....HR				WORKOUT	○ YES ○ NO
THU	Eating Window			NUMBER OF MEALS	SUGAR	○ YES ○ NO
					COFFEE	○ YES ○ NO
					WATER	○ YES ○ NO
FASTING TIME	○○○○○○○○○○○○○○○○○○○○○○○○ ....HR				WORKOUT	○ YES ○ NO
FRI	Eating Window			NUMBER OF MEALS	SUGAR	○ YES ○ NO
					COFFEE	○ YES ○ NO
					WATER	○ YES ○ NO
FASTING TIME	○○○○○○○○○○○○○○○○○○○○○○○○ ....HR				WORKOUT	○ YES ○ NO

NOTES & ACCOMPLISHMENT

DATA:		FASTING TIME TRACKER			

SAT
- Eating Window
- NUMBER OF MEALS:
- SUGAR ○ YES ○ NO
- COFFEE ○ YES ○ NO
- WATER ○ YES ○ NO

FASTING TIME: ○○○○○○○○○○○○○○○○○○○○○○○○ ....HR
WORKOUT ○ YES ○ NO

SUN
- Eating Window
- NUMBER OF MEALS:
- SUGAR ○ YES ○ NO
- COFFEE ○ YES ○ NO
- WATER ○ YES ○ NO

FASTING TIME: ○○○○○○○○○○○○○○○○○○○○○○○○ ....HR
WORKOUT ○ YES ○ NO

ENERGY LEVEL

SUN	MON	TUE	WED	THU	FRI	SAT

OBSERVATIONS - HOW I FEEL

MY GOAL THIS WEEK

MEASUREMENT:

CHEST................ WAIST................ HIPS................

WEIGHT:

DATA:		FASTING TIME TRACKER			
MON	Eating Window		NUMBER OF MEALS	SUGAR	○ YES ○ NO
				COFFEE	○ YES ○ NO
				WATER	○ YES ○ NO
FASTING TIME	○○○○○○○○○○○○○○○○○○○○○○○○		....HR	WORKOUT	○ YES ○ NO
TUE	Eating Window		NUMBER OF MEALS	SUGAR	○ YES ○ NO
				COFFEE	○ YES ○ NO
				WATER	○ YES ○ NO
FASTING TIME	○○○○○○○○○○○○○○○○○○○○○○○○		....HR	WORKOUT	○ YES ○ NO
WED	Eating Window		NUMBER OF MEALS	SUGAR	○ YES ○ NO
				COFFEE	○ YES ○ NO
				WATER	○ YES ○ NO
FASTING TIME	○○○○○○○○○○○○○○○○○○○○○○○○		....HR	WORKOUT	○ YES ○ NO
THU	Eating Window		NUMBER OF MEALS	SUGAR	○ YES ○ NO
				COFFEE	○ YES ○ NO
				WATER	○ YES ○ NO
FASTING TIME	○○○○○○○○○○○○○○○○○○○○○○○○		....HR	WORKOUT	○ YES ○ NO
FRI	Eating Window		NUMBER OF MEALS	SUGAR	○ YES ○ NO
				COFFEE	○ YES ○ NO
				WATER	○ YES ○ NO
FASTING TIME	○○○○○○○○○○○○○○○○○○○○○○○○		....HR	WORKOUT	○ YES ○ NO

NOTES & ACCOMPLISHMENT

DATA:		FASTING TIME TRACKER			

SAT	Eating Window	NUMBER OF MEALS	SUGAR ○YES ○NO
			COFFEE ○YES ○NO
			WATER ○YES ○NO
FASTING TIME	○○○○○○○○○○○○○○○○○○○○○○○○ H.R		WORKOUT ○YES ○NO
SUN	Eating Window	NUMBER OF MEALS	SUGAR ○YES ○NO
			COFFEE ○YES ○NO
			WATER ○YES ○NO
FASTING TIME	○○○○○○○○○○○○○○○○○○○○○○○○ H.R		WORKOUT ○YES ○NO

ENERGY LEVEL

SUN	MON	TUE	WED	THU	FRI	SAT

OBSERVATIONS - HOW I FEEL

MY GOAL THIS WEEK

MEASUREMENT:

WEIGHT:

CHEST................ WAIST................ HIPS................

FASTING TIME TRACKER

DATA: _____

MON
- Eating Window:
- NUMBER OF MEALS:
- SUGAR: ○ YES ○ NO
- COFFEE: ○ YES ○ NO
- WATER: ○ YES ○ NO
- FASTING TIME: .... H:R
- WORKOUT: ○ YES ○ NO

TUE
- Eating Window:
- NUMBER OF MEALS:
- SUGAR: ○ YES ○ NO
- COFFEE: ○ YES ○ NO
- WATER: ○ YES ○ NO
- FASTING TIME: .... H:R
- WORKOUT: ○ YES ○ NO

WED
- Eating Window:
- NUMBER OF MEALS:
- SUGAR: ○ YES ○ NO
- COFFEE: ○ YES ○ NO
- WATER: ○ YES ○ NO
- FASTING TIME: .... H:R
- WORKOUT: ○ YES ○ NO

THU
- Eating Window:
- NUMBER OF MEALS:
- SUGAR: ○ YES ○ NO
- COFFEE: ○ YES ○ NO
- WATER: ○ YES ○ NO
- FASTING TIME: .... H:R
- WORKOUT: ○ YES ○ NO

FRI
- Eating Window:
- NUMBER OF MEALS:
- SUGAR: ○ YES ○ NO
- COFFEE: ○ YES ○ NO
- WATER: ○ YES ○ NO
- FASTING TIME: .... H:R
- WORKOUT: ○ YES ○ NO

NOTES & ACCOMPLISHMENT

DATA:		FASTING TIME TRACKER			

SAT
- Eating Window
- NUMBER OF MEALS
- SUGAR ○ YES ○ NO
- COFFEE ○ YES ○ NO
- WATER ○ YES ○ NO

FASTING TIME: .... HR — WORKOUT ○ YES ○ NO

SUN
- Eating Window
- NUMBER OF MEALS
- SUGAR ○ YES ○ NO
- COFFEE ○ YES ○ NO
- WATER ○ YES ○ NO

FASTING TIME: .... HR — WORKOUT ○ YES ○ NO

ENERGY LEVEL

SUN	MON	TUE	WED	THU	FRI	SAT

OBSERVATIONS - HOW I FEEL

MY GOAL THIS WEEK

MEASUREMENT:

CHEST.............. WAIST.............. HIPS..............

WEIGHT:

DATA:		FASTING TIME TRACKER			
MON	Eating Window		NUMBER OF MEALS	SUGAR	◯ YES ◯ NO
				COFFEE	◯ YES ◯ NO
				WATER	◯ YES ◯ NO
FASTING TIME	◯◯◯◯◯◯◯◯◯◯◯◯◯◯◯◯◯◯◯◯◯◯◯◯		......HR	WORKOUT	◯ YES ◯ NO
TUE	Eating Window		NUMBER OF MEALS	SUGAR	◯ YES ◯ NO
				COFFEE	◯ YES ◯ NO
				WATER	◯ YES ◯ NO
FASTING TIME	◯◯◯◯◯◯◯◯◯◯◯◯◯◯◯◯◯◯◯◯◯◯◯◯		......HR	WORKOUT	◯ YES ◯ NO
WED	Eating Window		NUMBER OF MEALS	SUGAR	◯ YES ◯ NO
				COFFEE	◯ YES ◯ NO
				WATER	◯ YES ◯ NO
FASTING TIME	◯◯◯◯◯◯◯◯◯◯◯◯◯◯◯◯◯◯◯◯◯◯◯◯		......HR	WORKOUT	◯ YES ◯ NO
THU	Eating Window		NUMBER OF MEALS	SUGAR	◯ YES ◯ NO
				COFFEE	◯ YES ◯ NO
				WATER	◯ YES ◯ NO
FASTING TIME	◯◯◯◯◯◯◯◯◯◯◯◯◯◯◯◯◯◯◯◯◯◯◯◯		......HR	WORKOUT	◯ YES ◯ NO
FRI	Eating Window		NUMBER OF MEALS	SUGAR	◯ YES ◯ NO
				COFFEE	◯ YES ◯ NO
				WATER	◯ YES ◯ NO
FASTING TIME	◯◯◯◯◯◯◯◯◯◯◯◯◯◯◯◯◯◯◯◯◯◯◯◯		......HR	WORKOUT	◯ YES ◯ NO

NOTES & ACCOMPLISHMENT

DATA:		FASTING TIME TRACKER			
SAT	Eating Window		NUMBER OF MEALS	SUGAR ○ YES ○ NO	
				COFFEE ○ YES ○ NO	
				WATER ○ YES ○ NO	
FASTING TIME	○○○○○○○○○○○○○○○○○○○○○○○○ ...HR			WORKOUT ○ YES ○ NO	
SUN	Eating Window		NUMBER OF MEALS	SUGAR ○ YES ○ NO	
				COFFEE ○ YES ○ NO	
				WATER ○ YES ○ NO	
FASTING TIME	○○○○○○○○○○○○○○○○○○○○○○○○ ...HR			WORKOUT ○ YES ○ NO	

ENERGY LEVEL

SUN	MON	TUE	WED	THU	FRI	SAT

OBSERVATIONS - HOW I FEEL

MY GOAL THIS WEEK

MEASUREMENT:

WEIGHT:

CHEST............... WAIST............... HIPS...............

DATA:		FASTING TIME TRACKER			
MON	Eating Window		NUMBER OF MEALS	SUGAR	⭘ YES ⭘ NO
				COFFEE	⭘ YES ⭘ NO
				WATER	⭘ YES ⭘ NO
FASTING TIME	⭘⭘⭘⭘⭘⭘⭘⭘⭘⭘⭘⭘☀⭘⭘⭘⭘⭘⭘⭘⭘⭘⭘⭘		:HR	WORKOUT	⭘ YES ⭘ NO
TUE	Eating Window		NUMBER OF MEALS	SUGAR	⭘ YES ⭘ NO
				COFFEE	⭘ YES ⭘ NO
				WATER	⭘ YES ⭘ NO
FASTING TIME	⭘⭘⭘⭘⭘⭘⭘⭘⭘⭘⭘⭘☀⭘⭘⭘⭘⭘⭘⭘⭘⭘⭘⭘		:HR	WORKOUT	⭘ YES ⭘ NO
WED	Eating Window		NUMBER OF MEALS	SUGAR	⭘ YES ⭘ NO
				COFFEE	⭘ YES ⭘ NO
				WATER	⭘ YES ⭘ NO
FASTING TIME	⭘⭘⭘⭘⭘⭘⭘⭘⭘⭘⭘⭘☀⭘⭘⭘⭘⭘⭘⭘⭘⭘⭘⭘		:HR	WORKOUT	⭘ YES ⭘ NO
THU	Eating Window		NUMBER OF MEALS	SUGAR	⭘ YES ⭘ NO
				COFFEE	⭘ YES ⭘ NO
				WATER	⭘ YES ⭘ NO
FASTING TIME	⭘⭘⭘⭘⭘⭘⭘⭘⭘⭘⭘⭘☀⭘⭘⭘⭘⭘⭘⭘⭘⭘⭘⭘		:HR	WORKOUT	⭘ YES ⭘ NO
FRI	Eating Window		NUMBER OF MEALS	SUGAR	⭘ YES ⭘ NO
				COFFEE	⭘ YES ⭘ NO
				WATER	⭘ YES ⭘ NO
FASTING TIME	⭘⭘⭘⭘⭘⭘⭘⭘⭘⭘⭘⭘☀⭘⭘⭘⭘⭘⭘⭘⭘⭘⭘⭘		:HR	WORKOUT	⭘ YES ⭘ NO

NOTES & ACCOMPLISHMENT

DATA:		FASTING TIME TRACKER			

	Eating Window	NUMBER OF MEALS	SUGAR ⚪YES ⚪NO
SAT			COFFEE ⚪YES ⚪NO
			WATER ⚪YES ⚪NO
FASTING TIME	○○○○○○○○○○○○☼○○○○○○○○○○○○ ....HR		WORKOUT ⚪YES ⚪NO
	Eating Window	NUMBER OF MEALS	SUGAR ⚪YES ⚪NO
SUN			COFFEE ⚪YES ⚪NO
			WATER ⚪YES ⚪NO
FASTING TIME	○○○○○○○○○○○○☼○○○○○○○○○○○○ ....HR		WORKOUT ⚪YES ⚪NO

ENERGY LEVEL

😊 🙂 😏 😯 😬 😵

SUN	MON	TUE	WED	THU	FRI	SAT

OBSERVATIONS - HOW I FEEL

MY GOAL THIS WEEK

MEASUREMENT:

CHEST.............. WAIST.............. HIPS..............

WEIGHT:

DATA:		FASTING TIME TRACKER			
MON	Eating Window		NUMBER OF MEALS	SUGAR	○ YES ○ NO
				COFFEE	○ YES ○ NO
				WATER	○ YES ○ NO
FASTING TIME	○○○○○○○○○○○○○○○○○○○○○○○○		....H:R	WORKOUT	○ YES ○ NO
TUE	Eating Window		NUMBER OF MEALS	SUGAR	○ YES ○ NO
				COFFEE	○ YES ○ NO
				WATER	○ YES ○ NO
FASTING TIME	○○○○○○○○○○○○○○○○○○○○○○○○		....H:R	WORKOUT	○ YES ○ NO
WED	Eating Window		NUMBER OF MEALS	SUGAR	○ YES ○ NO
				COFFEE	○ YES ○ NO
				WATER	○ YES ○ NO
FASTING TIME	○○○○○○○○○○○○○○○○○○○○○○○○		....H:R	WORKOUT	○ YES ○ NO
THU	Eating Window		NUMBER OF MEALS	SUGAR	○ YES ○ NO
				COFFEE	○ YES ○ NO
				WATER	○ YES ○ NO
FASTING TIME	○○○○○○○○○○○○○○○○○○○○○○○○		....H:R	WORKOUT	○ YES ○ NO
FRI	Eating Window		NUMBER OF MEALS	SUGAR	○ YES ○ NO
				COFFEE	○ YES ○ NO
				WATER	○ YES ○ NO
FASTING TIME	○○○○○○○○○○○○○○○○○○○○○○○○		....H:R	WORKOUT	○ YES ○ NO

NOTES & ACCOMPLISHMENT

| DATA: | | | | FASTING TIME TRACKER | | | | |

SAT

Eating Window		NUMBER OF MEALS	SUGAR ○ YES ○ NO
			COFFEE ○ YES ○ NO
			WATER ○ YES ○ NO

FASTING TIME ○○○○○○○○○○○○○○○○○○○○○○○○ ....HR   WORKOUT ○ YES ○ NO

SUN

Eating Window		NUMBER OF MEALS	SUGAR ○ YES ○ NO
			COFFEE ○ YES ○ NO
			WATER ○ YES ○ NO

FASTING TIME ○○○○○○○○○○○○○○○○○○○○○○○○ ....HR   WORKOUT ○ YES ○ NO

ENERGY LEVEL

😄 🙂 😏 😮 😬 😟

SUN	MON	TUE	WED	THU	FRI	SAT

OBSERVATIONS - HOW I FEEL

MY GOAL THIS WEEK

MEASUREMENT:

CHEST............ WAIST............ HIPS............

WEIGHT:

DATA: _____   **FASTING TIME TRACKER**

	Eating Window	NUMBER OF MEALS	SUGAR ○YES ○NO
MON			COFFEE ○YES ○NO
			WATER ○YES ○NO
FASTING TIME	○○○○○○○○○○○○○○○○○○○○○○○○ ....HR		WORKOUT ○YES ○NO
TUE	Eating Window	NUMBER OF MEALS	SUGAR ○YES ○NO
			COFFEE ○YES ○NO
			WATER ○YES ○NO
FASTING TIME	○○○○○○○○○○○○○○○○○○○○○○○○ ....HR		WORKOUT ○YES ○NO
WED	Eating Window	NUMBER OF MEALS	SUGAR ○YES ○NO
			COFFEE ○YES ○NO
			WATER ○YES ○NO
FASTING TIME	○○○○○○○○○○○○○○○○○○○○○○○○ ....HR		WORKOUT ○YES ○NO
THU	Eating Window	NUMBER OF MEALS	SUGAR ○YES ○NO
			COFFEE ○YES ○NO
			WATER ○YES ○NO
FASTING TIME	○○○○○○○○○○○○○○○○○○○○○○○○ ....HR		WORKOUT ○YES ○NO
FRI	Eating Window	NUMBER OF MEALS	SUGAR ○YES ○NO
			COFFEE ○YES ○NO
			WATER ○YES ○NO
FASTING TIME	○○○○○○○○○○○○○○○○○○○○○○○○ ....HR		WORKOUT ○YES ○NO

NOTES & ACCOMPLISHMENT

DATA:			FASTING TIME TRACKER			

SAT
- Eating Window
- NUMBER OF MEALS
- SUGAR ○ YES ○ NO
- COFFEE ○ YES ○ NO
- WATER ○ YES ○ NO
- FASTING TIME ....HR
- WORKOUT ○ YES ○ NO

SUN
- Eating Window
- NUMBER OF MEALS
- SUGAR ○ YES ○ NO
- COFFEE ○ YES ○ NO
- WATER ○ YES ○ NO
- FASTING TIME ....HR
- WORKOUT ○ YES ○ NO

ENERGY LEVEL

SUN	MON	TUE	WED	THU	FRI	SAT

OBSERVATIONS - HOW I FEEL

MY GOAL THIS WEEK

MEASUREMENT:

CHEST................ WAIST................ HIPS................

WEIGHT:

DATA:	FASTING TIME TRACKER		

MON
Eating Window | NUMBER OF MEALS
SUGAR ○ YES ○ NO
COFFEE ○ YES ○ NO
WATER ○ YES ○ NO

FASTING TIME ......HR | WORKOUT ○ YES ○ NO

TUE
Eating Window | NUMBER OF MEALS
SUGAR ○ YES ○ NO
COFFEE ○ YES ○ NO
WATER ○ YES ○ NO

FASTING TIME ......HR | WORKOUT ○ YES ○ NO

WED
Eating Window | NUMBER OF MEALS
SUGAR ○ YES ○ NO
COFFEE ○ YES ○ NO
WATER ○ YES ○ NO

FASTING TIME ......HR | WORKOUT ○ YES ○ NO

THU
Eating Window | NUMBER OF MEALS
SUGAR ○ YES ○ NO
COFFEE ○ YES ○ NO
WATER ○ YES ○ NO

FASTING TIME ......HR | WORKOUT ○ YES ○ NO

FRI
Eating Window | NUMBER OF MEALS
SUGAR ○ YES ○ NO
COFFEE ○ YES ○ NO
WATER ○ YES ○ NO

FASTING TIME ......HR | WORKOUT ○ YES ○ NO

NOTES & ACCOMPLISHMENT

DATA:		FASTING TIME TRACKER			

SAT
- Eating Window
- NUMBER OF MEALS
- SUGAR ○ YES ○ NO
- COFFEE ○ YES ○ NO
- WATER ○ YES ○ NO
- FASTING TIME .... HR
- WORKOUT ○ YES ○ NO

SUN
- Eating Window
- NUMBER OF MEALS
- SUGAR ○ YES ○ NO
- COFFEE ○ YES ○ NO
- WATER ○ YES ○ NO
- FASTING TIME .... HR
- WORKOUT ○ YES ○ NO

ENERGY LEVEL

SUN	MON	TUE	WED	THU	FRI	SAT

OBSERVATIONS - HOW I FEEL

MY GOAL THIS WEEK

MEASUREMENT:

CHEST................ WAIST................ HIPS................

WEIGHT:

FASTING TIME TRACKER

DATA: _____

MON
Eating Window:

NUMBER OF MEALS:

SUGAR ○ YES ○ NO
COFFEE ○ YES ○ NO
WATER ○ YES ○ NO

FASTING TIME: .... HR

WORKOUT ○ YES ○ NO

TUE
Eating Window:

NUMBER OF MEALS:

SUGAR ○ YES ○ NO
COFFEE ○ YES ○ NO
WATER ○ YES ○ NO

FASTING TIME: .... HR

WORKOUT ○ YES ○ NO

WED
Eating Window:

NUMBER OF MEALS:

SUGAR ○ YES ○ NO
COFFEE ○ YES ○ NO
WATER ○ YES ○ NO

FASTING TIME: .... HR

WORKOUT ○ YES ○ NO

THU
Eating Window:

NUMBER OF MEALS:

SUGAR ○ YES ○ NO
COFFEE ○ YES ○ NO
WATER ○ YES ○ NO

FASTING TIME: .... HR

WORKOUT ○ YES ○ NO

FRI
Eating Window:

NUMBER OF MEALS:

SUGAR ○ YES ○ NO
COFFEE ○ YES ○ NO
WATER ○ YES ○ NO

FASTING TIME: .... HR

WORKOUT ○ YES ○ NO

NOTES & ACCOMPLISHMENT

DATA:		FASTING TIME TRACKER			

SAT
- Eating Window
- NUMBER OF MEALS
- SUGAR ○ YES ○ NO
- COFFEE ○ YES ○ NO
- WATER ○ YES ○ NO
- FASTING TIME ....HR
- WORKOUT ○ YES ○ NO

SUN
- Eating Window
- NUMBER OF MEALS
- SUGAR ○ YES ○ NO
- COFFEE ○ YES ○ NO
- WATER ○ YES ○ NO
- FASTING TIME ....HR
- WORKOUT ○ YES ○ NO

ENERGY LEVEL

SUN	MON	TUE	WED	THU	FRI	SAT

OBSERVATIONS - HOW I FEEL

MY GOAL THIS WEEK

MEASUREMENT:

CHEST.......... WAIST.......... HIPS..........

WEIGHT:

DATA:		FASTING TIME TRACKER		

MON	Eating Window	NUMBER OF MEALS	SUGAR ⭘ YES ⭘ NO
			COFFEE ⭘ YES ⭘ NO
			WATER ⭘ YES ⭘ NO
FASTING TIME	⭘⭘⭘⭘⭘⭘⭘⭘⭘⭘⭘⭘⭘⭘⭘⭘⭘⭘⭘⭘⭘⭘⭘⭘ ....HR		WORKOUT ⭘ YES ⭘ NO

TUE	Eating Window	NUMBER OF MEALS	SUGAR ⭘ YES ⭘ NO
			COFFEE ⭘ YES ⭘ NO
			WATER ⭘ YES ⭘ NO
FASTING TIME	⭘⭘⭘⭘⭘⭘⭘⭘⭘⭘⭘⭘⭘⭘⭘⭘⭘⭘⭘⭘⭘⭘⭘⭘ ....HR		WORKOUT ⭘ YES ⭘ NO

WED	Eating Window	NUMBER OF MEALS	SUGAR ⭘ YES ⭘ NO
			COFFEE ⭘ YES ⭘ NO
			WATER ⭘ YES ⭘ NO
FASTING TIME	⭘⭘⭘⭘⭘⭘⭘⭘⭘⭘⭘⭘⭘⭘⭘⭘⭘⭘⭘⭘⭘⭘⭘⭘ ....HR		WORKOUT ⭘ YES ⭘ NO

THU	Eating Window	NUMBER OF MEALS	SUGAR ⭘ YES ⭘ NO
			COFFEE ⭘ YES ⭘ NO
			WATER ⭘ YES ⭘ NO
FASTING TIME	⭘⭘⭘⭘⭘⭘⭘⭘⭘⭘⭘⭘⭘⭘⭘⭘⭘⭘⭘⭘⭘⭘⭘⭘ ....HR		WORKOUT ⭘ YES ⭘ NO

FRI	Eating Window	NUMBER OF MEALS	SUGAR ⭘ YES ⭘ NO
			COFFEE ⭘ YES ⭘ NO
			WATER ⭘ YES ⭘ NO
FASTING TIME	⭘⭘⭘⭘⭘⭘⭘⭘⭘⭘⭘⭘⭘⭘⭘⭘⭘⭘⭘⭘⭘⭘⭘⭘ ....HR		WORKOUT ⭘ YES ⭘ NO

NOTES & ACCOMPLISHMENT

DATA:		FASTING TIME TRACKER			

SAT

Eating Window	NUMBER OF MEALS	SUGAR ◯ YES ◯ NO
		COFFEE ◯ YES ◯ NO
		WATER ◯ YES ◯ NO

FASTING TIME: ◯◯◯◯◯◯◯◯◯◯◯◯◯◯◯◯◯◯◯◯◯◯◯◯ ....HR **WORKOUT** ◯ YES ◯ NO

SUN

Eating Window	NUMBER OF MEALS	SUGAR ◯ YES ◯ NO
		COFFEE ◯ YES ◯ NO
		WATER ◯ YES ◯ NO

FASTING TIME: ◯◯◯◯◯◯◯◯◯◯◯◯◯◯◯◯◯◯◯◯◯◯◯◯ ....HR **WORKOUT** ◯ YES ◯ NO

ENERGY LEVEL

😊 🙂 😏 😮 😁 😬

SUN	MON	TUE	WED	THU	FRI	SAT

OBSERVATIONS - HOW I FEEL

MY GOAL THIS WEEK

MEASUREMENT:

CHEST................ WAIST................ HIPS................

WEIGHT:

| DATA: | | FASTING TIME TRACKER | | |

MON
Eating Window | NUMBER OF MEALS
SUGAR ○ YES ○ NO
COFFEE ○ YES ○ NO
WATER ○ YES ○ NO
FASTING TIME: ....HR — WORKOUT ○ YES ○ NO

TUE
Eating Window | NUMBER OF MEALS
SUGAR ○ YES ○ NO
COFFEE ○ YES ○ NO
WATER ○ YES ○ NO
FASTING TIME: ....HR — WORKOUT ○ YES ○ NO

WED
Eating Window | NUMBER OF MEALS
SUGAR ○ YES ○ NO
COFFEE ○ YES ○ NO
WATER ○ YES ○ NO
FASTING TIME: ....HR — WORKOUT ○ YES ○ NO

THU
Eating Window | NUMBER OF MEALS
SUGAR ○ YES ○ NO
COFFEE ○ YES ○ NO
WATER ○ YES ○ NO
FASTING TIME: ....HR — WORKOUT ○ YES ○ NO

FRI
Eating Window | NUMBER OF MEALS
SUGAR ○ YES ○ NO
COFFEE ○ YES ○ NO
WATER ○ YES ○ NO
FASTING TIME: ....HR — WORKOUT ○ YES ○ NO

NOTES & ACCOMPLISHMENT

DATA:		**FASTING TIME TRACKER**			

SAT	Eating Window	NUMBER OF MEALS	SUGAR ⊙ YES ⊙ NO
			COFFEE ⊙ YES ⊙ NO
			WATER ⊙ YES ⊙ NO
FASTING TIME	○○○○○○○○○○○○○○○○○○○○○○○○ ....HR		WORKOUT ⊙ YES ⊙ NO

SUN	Eating Window	NUMBER OF MEALS	SUGAR ⊙ YES ⊙ NO
			COFFEE ⊙ YES ⊙ NO
			WATER ⊙ YES ⊙ NO
FASTING TIME	○○○○○○○○○○○○○○○○○○○○○○○○ ....HR		WORKOUT ⊙ YES ⊙ NO

ENERGY LEVEL

SUN	MON	TUE	WED	THU	FRI	SAT

OBSERVATIONS - HOW I FEEL

MY GOAL THIS WEEK

MEASUREMENT:

CHEST.................... WAIST.................... HIPS....................

WEIGHT:

DATA:		FASTING TIME TRACKER			
MON	Eating Window		NUMBER OF MEALS	SUGAR	○ YES ○ NO
				COFFEE	○ YES ○ NO
				WATER	○ YES ○ NO
FASTING TIME	○○○○○○○○○○○○○○○○○○○○○○○○		......HR	WORKOUT	○ YES ○ NO
TUE	Eating Window		NUMBER OF MEALS	SUGAR	○ YES ○ NO
				COFFEE	○ YES ○ NO
				WATER	○ YES ○ NO
FASTING TIME	○○○○○○○○○○○○○○○○○○○○○○○○		......HR	WORKOUT	○ YES ○ NO
WED	Eating Window		NUMBER OF MEALS	SUGAR	○ YES ○ NO
				COFFEE	○ YES ○ NO
				WATER	○ YES ○ NO
FASTING TIME	○○○○○○○○○○○○○○○○○○○○○○○○		......HR	WORKOUT	○ YES ○ NO
THU	Eating Window		NUMBER OF MEALS	SUGAR	○ YES ○ NO
				COFFEE	○ YES ○ NO
				WATER	○ YES ○ NO
FASTING TIME	○○○○○○○○○○○○○○○○○○○○○○○○		......HR	WORKOUT	○ YES ○ NO
FRI	Eating Window		NUMBER OF MEALS	SUGAR	○ YES ○ NO
				COFFEE	○ YES ○ NO
				WATER	○ YES ○ NO
FASTING TIME	○○○○○○○○○○○○○○○○○○○○○○○○		......HR	WORKOUT	○ YES ○ NO

NOTES & ACCOMPLISHMENT

DATA:		FASTING TIME TRACKER			

SAT
- Eating Window:
- Number of Meals:
- Sugar: ○ YES ○ NO
- Coffee: ○ YES ○ NO
- Water: ○ YES ○ NO
- Fasting Time: ___ HR
- Workout: ○ YES ○ NO

SUN
- Eating Window:
- Number of Meals:
- Sugar: ○ YES ○ NO
- Coffee: ○ YES ○ NO
- Water: ○ YES ○ NO
- Fasting Time: ___ HR
- Workout: ○ YES ○ NO

ENERGY LEVEL

SUN	MON	TUE	WED	THU	FRI	SAT

OBSERVATIONS - HOW I FEEL

MY GOAL THIS WEEK

MEASUREMENT:

CHEST............ WAIST............ HIPS............

WEIGHT:

DATA:	FASTING TIME TRACKER		

MON
Eating Window

NUMBER OF MEALS

SUGAR	◯ YES ◯ NO
COFFEE	◯ YES ◯ NO
WATER	◯ YES ◯ NO

FASTING TIME ....H:R WORKOUT ◯ YES ◯ NO

TUE
Eating Window

NUMBER OF MEALS

SUGAR	◯ YES ◯ NO
COFFEE	◯ YES ◯ NO
WATER	◯ YES ◯ NO

FASTING TIME ....H:R WORKOUT ◯ YES ◯ NO

WED
Eating Window

NUMBER OF MEALS

SUGAR	◯ YES ◯ NO
COFFEE	◯ YES ◯ NO
WATER	◯ YES ◯ NO

FASTING TIME ....H:R WORKOUT ◯ YES ◯ NO

THU
Eating Window

NUMBER OF MEALS

SUGAR	◯ YES ◯ NO
COFFEE	◯ YES ◯ NO
WATER	◯ YES ◯ NO

FASTING TIME ....H:R WORKOUT ◯ YES ◯ NO

FRI
Eating Window

NUMBER OF MEALS

SUGAR	◯ YES ◯ NO
COFFEE	◯ YES ◯ NO
WATER	◯ YES ◯ NO

FASTING TIME ....H:R WORKOUT ◯ YES ◯ NO

NOTES & ACCOMPLISHMENT

DATA:		FASTING TIME TRACKER		

SAT
- Eating Window
- NUMBER OF MEALS:
- SUGAR ○ YES ○ NO
- COFFEE ○ YES ○ NO
- WATER ○ YES ○ NO

FASTING TIME: ○○○○○○○○○○○○○○○○○○○○○○○○ ......HR WORKOUT ○ YES ○ NO

SUN
- Eating Window
- NUMBER OF MEALS:
- SUGAR ○ YES ○ NO
- COFFEE ○ YES ○ NO
- WATER ○ YES ○ NO

FASTING TIME: ○○○○○○○○○○○○○○○○○○○○○○○○ ......HR WORKOUT ○ YES ○ NO

ENERGY LEVEL

SUN	MON	TUE	WED	THU	FRI	SAT

OBSERVATIONS - HOW I FEEL

MY GOAL THIS WEEK

MEASUREMENT:

CHEST................ WAIST................ HIPS................

WEIGHT:

Made in United States
North Haven, CT
06 June 2025